2020 GLUTEN FREE BUYERS GUIDE

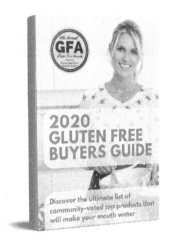

JOSH SCHIEFFER

Table of Contents

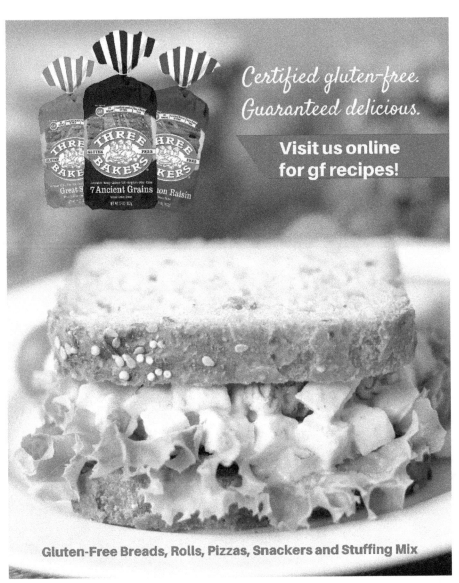

Introduction by Josh Schieffer

First, let me thank you for picking up this book. We are delighted you have decided to find the best in gluten-free. This book has been carefully designed to help you quickly connect with the best gluten-free products, people, services, and organizations. We host the Annual Gluten-Free Awards; a program that enables the gluten-free community to cast votes for their favorites. This year we had 3,937 people take part in the voting process. The 117,874 individual responses are all rolled up in the following pages.

This year we changed the cover design and added a few new gluten free award categories now totaling 61!

HOW THE GLUTEN FREE AWARDS WORK

Presented by The Gluten Free Buyers Guide

PRODUCT REGISTRATION

Gluten Free Buyers Guide Registration

Each year brands register their products in The Gluten Free Buyers Guide. The guide consists of 60 gluten free categories ranging from gluten free bread to gluten free comfort food. Find more registration details at GlutenFreeBuyersGuide.com

GLUTEN FREE BLOGGERS & INFLUENCERS

Top bloggers & influences register products

We generate a list of 20-30 top gluten free bloggers and social media influencers. We ask them to register their favorite brands and products to be submitted into The Gluten Free Buyers Guide.

COMMUNITY VOTE

We ask the gluten free community to vote

Once we have the products registered for The Gluten Free Buyers Guide we create a voting ballot with those products listed in their respected categories. Nearly 10,000 people in the gluten free community vote for their favorites.

PUBLISHING

We publish The Gluten Free Buyers Guide

The Gluten Free Buyers Guide publishes all products that had been registered highlighting the top three GFA Award Winners in each category. The winners will have an image of their product so consumers can quickly identify those products while shopping

Our Story

The story behind The Gluten Free Awards that very few people know

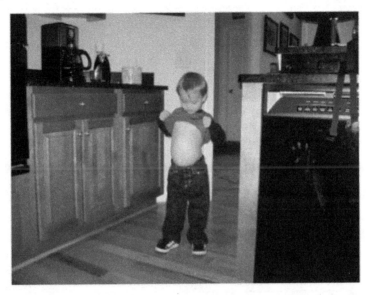

I remember it like it was yesterday when my four-year-old son Jacob, now fifteen, was playing in the kiddie pool with other kids that I assumed were his age based on their height. After asking all the surrounding kids what ages they were, I realized Jacob was significantly smaller than kids his own age. This prompted my wife and I to seek a professional opinion. After consulting with our family physician, she confirmed that Jacob had essentially stopped growing for an entire year without us realizing it. He was referred to Jeff Gordon's Children's Hospital in Charlotte North Carolina to discuss possible growth hormone therapy. The doctors there reviewed Jacob's case and requested a few blood tests based on some suspicions they had.

Our cell phone service at our house was terrible so when the doctor finally called with the blood results, my wife and I ran to the front of the driveway to hear the doctor clearly. With a sporadic signal, we heard "Jacob has celiac disease." We looked at each other as tears ran down my wife's face. We huddled closer to the phone and asked, "what is celiac disease?". After getting a brief description mixed with crappy cell service and happy neighbors waving as they drove by, my wife and I embraced and wept. We were told to maintain his normal diet until we could have an endoscopy and biopsy for further confirmation. Once confirmed our next visit was to a registered dietitian for guidance.

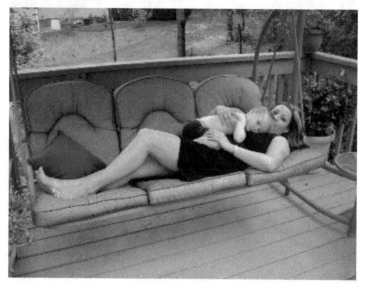

Jayme, my wife, made the appointment and called me with a weird request. "Will you meet me at the dietitian's house for a consultation?". I was confused when she said to go to her house. Jayme then explained that the dietician's daughter had celiac disease too and the best way to show the new lifestyle to patients would be to dive right in. I'll admit, it was a bit uncomfortable at first to be in a strangers' house looking at their personal items but looking back now, I wouldn't change it for the world. That encounter is ultimately the motivation behind The Gluten Free Awards and the associated Gluten Free Buyers Guide. We left her house with complete understanding of cross contamination, best practices and what products they personally liked and disliked. That visit was life changing and left us feeling confident as we made our way to the local health food store.

That first trip shopping took forever. Each label was read, and cross checked with our list of known gluten containing suspects. It was also shocking to see the bill when it was time to pay. We had replaced our entire pantry and fridge with all products that had the "Gluten Free" label. We both worked full-time and had decent paying jobs and it still set us back financially.

We looked for support groups locally and came across a "100% Gluten-Free Picnic" in Raleigh, which was two hours away from where we lived. This was our first time meeting other people with celiac disease and we were fortunate to have met some informative people that were willing to help with the hundreds of questions we had. We were introduced to a family whose son had been recently diagnosed with celiac disease as well. His condition was much worse than Jacobs and he was almost hospitalized before finally being diagnosed. They confided in us as we shared similar stories. There were two differences that would change my life forever. The first was the fact that they didn't have the same experience with a registered dietitian. Instead they were handed a two-page Xerox copy of "safe foods". Second, they didn't have the financial security to experiment with gluten free counterparts. Their first two months exposed to the gluten free lifestyle left them extremely depressed and broke.

On our way home from that picnic, Jayme and I felt compelled to help make a difference in some way. We were determined to help that family and others being diagnosed with this disease. Up until that day, we hadn't found a resource that gave unbiased opinions on gluten free products and services. Fast forward a few years and I too was diagnosed with celiac disease. That year, The Gluten Free Awards were born.

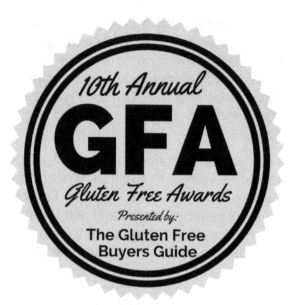

Originally our vision was to create a one-page website with a handful of categories organized by peoples' favorites. Since 2010 we have produced The Annual Gluten Free Awards (GFA) growing into sixty gluten free categories. After several requests, in 2014, we took the GFA results and published our first Gluten Free Buyers Guide. The annual guide is sold primarily in the United States however we continue to see increased global sales. Each year we have over 3,000 people vote for their favorite gluten free products and we now communicate to nearly 21,000 people weekly through our email list.

We want to thank those special people and organizations that brought us to where we are today:

Pat Fogarty MS, RD, LDN for allowing us to enter your home.

Jeff Gordon's Children's Hospital

Raleigh Celiac Support Groups

Dean Meisel, MD, FAAP for the excellent medical care he provides for our family.

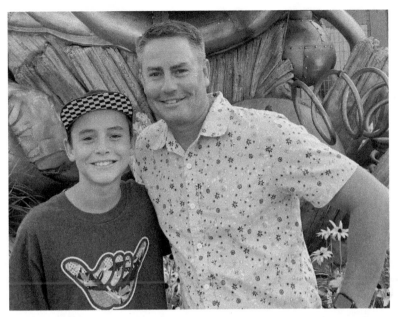

I hope you have learned something new from the story behind The Gluten Free Awards. Today, Jacob and I continue to live a healthy gluten free lifestyle.

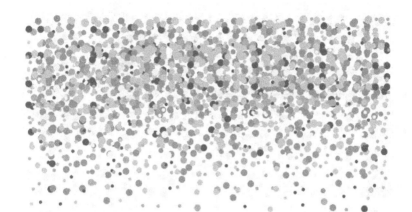

Celebrating 10 Years of connecting the gluten free community to the best products, people and services. THANK YOU!

Best Gluten Free Bagels

10th Annual Gluten-Free Awards:

1st Place Winner: Canyon Bakehouse Everything Bagels

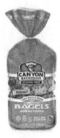

2nd Place Winner: ALDI: liveGfree Gluten Free Bagels - Plain

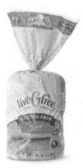

3rd Place Winner: Canyon Bakehouse Cinnamon Raisin Bagel

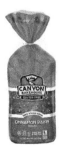

Other Great Products:

Udi's Cinnamon Raisin Bagels

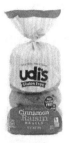

Canyon Bakehouse Blueberry Bagel

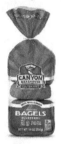

New Cascadia Traditional Sesame Bagels

The Greater Knead - Plain

CELIAC SURVEY

We polled over 400 people with celiac disease with the intent to make you feel not so alone.

How long have you had Celiac Disease?

Average length: 15 years

6,695 combined years of experience

Presented by The 2020 Gluten Free Buyers Guide

YOU'RE NOT ALONE

Best Gluten Free Beer Brands

10th Annual Gluten-Free Awards:

1st Place Winner: Redbridge

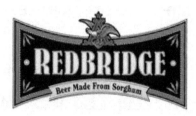

2nd Place Winner: Glutenberg

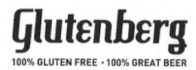

3rd Place Winner: Ghostfish Brewing Company

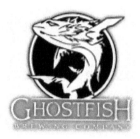

Other Great Products:

Bard's

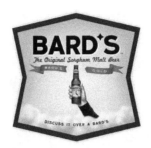

Ground Breaker Brewing

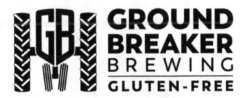

Holidaily Brewing

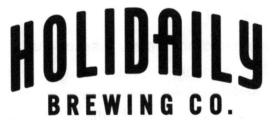

Alt Brew

Divine Science Brewing

Meet Christina Kantzavelos

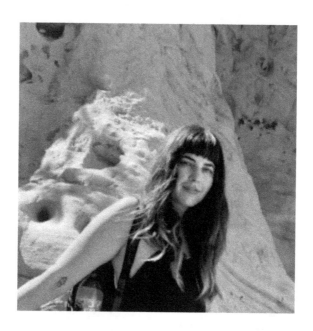

How long have you been gluten free?

Since 2012

Do you have any other dietary restrictions?

Dairy (casein), alcohol, soy, refined sugar, and a few high-histamine foods.

What has been your biggest challenge thus far?

As my food intolerances have increased, it's been challenging to purchase meals at restaurants (even with dedicated kitchens) without having to ask for a complete ingredients list and making alterations. I often have to ask for sides of everything and create my meals that way.

Where is your favorite place to eat?

My kitchen (my restrictions do not restrict me from getting extremely creative with what I make). Otherwise, there are a few dedicated restaurants here in San Diego that I love and trust.

Do you have any gluten related pet peeves?

The fact that it often gets confused with veganism. Or, that many people assume that if it's gluten-free it's automatically safe for us to eat. Hello, cross-contact!

Do you have any relatives are close friends that are gluten free?

Quite a few! It definitely makes me feel less alone.

Do you have a gluten horror story?

I don't have any true 'horror stories,' however, accidentally ingesting something due to cross-contact and/or lack of communication has led to some very uncomfortable moments, both physically and emotionally. For that reason, I use my gluten-sensor whenever I question something I'm about to eat. I've also learned to carry snacks with me wherever I go since I never truly know what the situation will look like upon arrival. I've attended past events where I was told I would have options, only to find out I didn't. That's pretty scary!

What has been the biggest change since you became gluten free?

I have felt so much healthier, overall. My symptoms were mitigated enough for me to not look back.

In ten years, a gluten free diet will be...

easier, safer, and streamlined.

What is the best advice you received?

"Getting your health back will taste better than anything with gluten in it." They were right.

What is the best way for people to connect with you?

Instagram - @buenqamino

Blog - www.buenqamino.com

Best Gluten Free Bloggers & Influencers

10th Annual Gluten-Free Awards:

Carol Kicinski from simplygluten-free.com

Carrie Veatch from forglutensake.com

Christina Kantzavelos from buenqamino.com

Chrystal Carver from glutenfreepalate.com

Dr. Alessio Fasano from massgeneral.org

Dr. Tom O'Bryan from thedr.com

Elana Amsterdam from elanaspantry.com

Elisabeth Hasselbeck from twitter.com/ehasselbeck

Erica Dermer from celiacandthebeast.com

Erin Smith from glutenfreeglobetrotter.com

Gluten Dude from glutendude.com

Hannah Crane from gfguru.org

Hayley Johnston from sociableceliac.com

Jackie Aanonsen McEwan from glutenfreefollowme.com

Jenna Drew from jennadrew.com

Jennifer Esposito from chewthis.life

Jessica Hanson from tastymeditation.com

Jillian Estell from jilliannicoleestell.com

Jules Shepherd from gfjules.com

Lori Miller from glutenfreeglobalicious.com

Matt Hansen from wheatlesswanderlust.com

Maureen Stanley from holdthegluten.com

Melinda Lawer Arcara from glutenfreebebe.com

Michael Frolichstein from celiacproject.com

Michelle Palin from mygluten-freekitchen.com

Nadine Grzeskowiak from glutenfreern.com

Nicole Hunn from glutenfreeonashoestring.com

Shay Lachendro from whattheforkfoodblog.com

Taylor Miller from halelifeblog.com

Tricia Thompson from glutenfreewatchdog.org

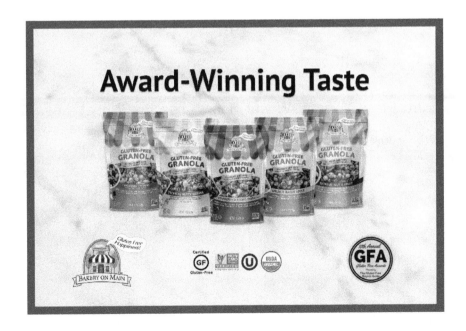

Best Gluten Free Books

10th Annual Gluten-Free Awards:

1st Place Winner: The First Year: Celiac Disease and Living Gluten-Free: An Essential Guide for the Newly Diagnosed: Jules Shepard

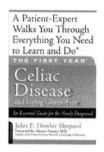

2nd Place Winner: Gluten Is My Bitch: Rants, Recipes, and Ridiculousness for the Gluten-Free by April Peveteaux

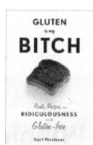

3rd Place Winner: Wheat Belly: Lose the Wheat, Lose the Weight, and Find Your Path Back to Health by William Davis

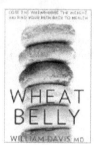

Other Great Books:

Jennifer's Way: My Journey with Celiac Disease--What Doctors Don't Tell You and How You Can Learn to Live Again by Jennifer Esposito

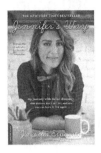

Celiac and the Beast: A Love Story Between a Gluten-Free Girl, Her Genes, and a Broken Digestive Tract by Erica Dermer

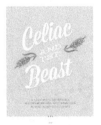

The Grain Brain Whole Life Plan: Boost Brain Performance, Lose Weight, and Achieve Optimal Health by Perlmutter MD, David and Kristin Loberg

Gluten Freedom: The Nation's Leading Expert Offers the Essential Guide to a Healthy, Gluten-Free Lifestyle by Alessio Fasano (Author), Susie Flaherty (Contributor)

3 Steps to Gluten-Free Living by Melinda Arcara

Dough Nation by Nadine Grzeskowiak

CELIAC SURVEY

We polled over 400 people with celiac disease with the intent to make you feel not so alone.

Have you helped anyone get diagnosed with Celiac Disease?

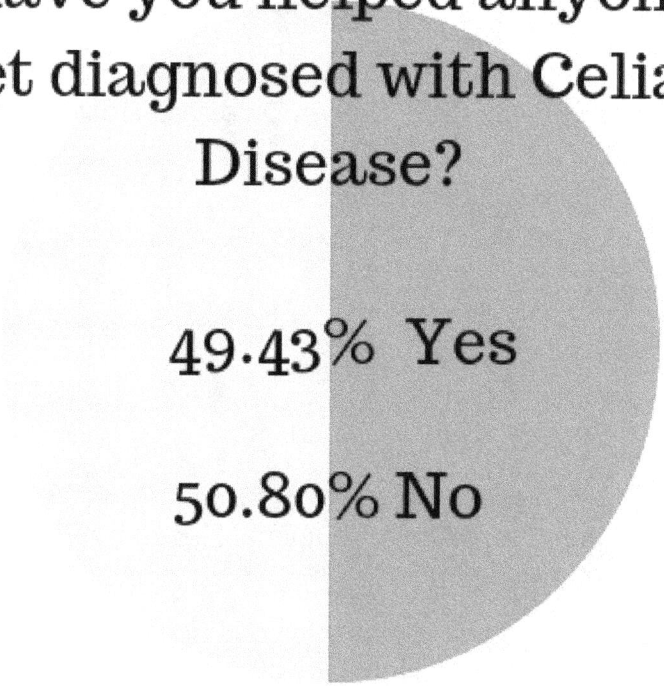

49.43% Yes

50.80% No

Presented by The 2020 Gluten Free Buyers Guide

YOU'RE NOT ALONE

Meet Jillian Estell

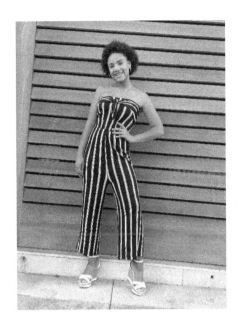

How long have you been gluten free?

15 years - my whole life

Do you have any other dietary restrictions?

No cashews, pistachios, dairy or corn

What has been your biggest challenge thus far?

Going out to eat

Where is your favorite place to eat?

Hillstone

Do you have any gluten related pet peeves?

Not really...maybe that people don't realize I can't have bread, crackers, pasta. etc..

Do you have any relatives are close friends that are gluten free?

My cousin is Celiac also

Do you have a gluten horror story?

I was served a regular sandwich and I ate half of it. We asked the restaurant several times to confirm it was gluten free. I was so sick and had to go to the ER and had side effects for 3 weeks.

What has been the biggest change since you became gluten free?

I've always been gluten free.

In ten years, a gluten free diet will be...

Very common

What is the best advice you received?

Bring your own food everywhere you go

What is the best way for people to connect with you?

Instagram @jillianestell

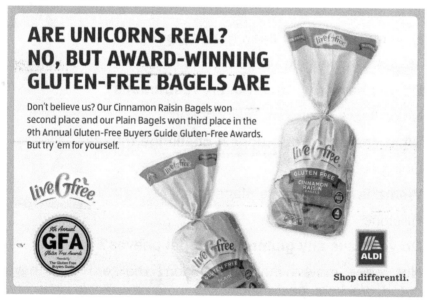

Best Gluten Free Bread Brands

10th Annual Gluten-Free Awards:

1st Place Winner: Canyon Bakehouse Heritage Honey White

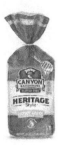

2nd Place Winner: Schar Deli Style Bread

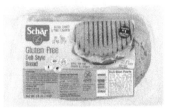

3rd Place Winner: Canyon Bakehouse 7-Grain Bread

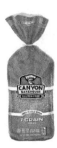

Other Great Products:

Canyon Bakehouse Ancient Grain Bread

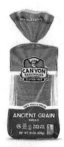

Three Bakers 7 Ancient Grains

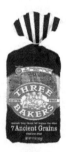

Three Bakers Whole Grain White

Mikey's Original English Muffin

Sweet PotaTOASTS, from the creators of CAULIPOWER - Roasted Sweet Potato Slices

Bread SRSLY Sourdough

Three Bakers Rye Style

Best Gluten Free Bread Crumbs

10th Annual Gluten-Free Awards:

1st Place Winner: Ian's Italian Panko Bread Crumbs

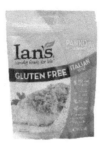

2nd Place Winner: 4C Seasoned Gluten Free Bread Crumbs

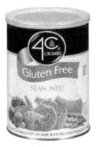

3rd Place Winner: Katz Gluten Free Bread Crumbs

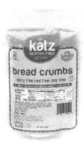

Yes, as a matter of fact, I do! It is irksome when people are told the wrong information about healing, the quality and nutrient density of the food matters, when celiac specialists don't declare conflicts of interest when talking about CD & NCGS and the false idea that someone will come up with a pill or vaccine that will allow people to eat gluten again. There is work to be done educating!

Do you have any relatives are close friends that are gluten free?

Yes, absolutely.

Do you have a gluten horror story?

Getting hit with gluten at the Columbia University Celiac Disease Center's conference. The venue that hosted the International Celiac Disease Symposium in Paris this year provided 'Gluten Free' lunches that contained wheat. These are just two examples. There are many more

What has been the biggest change since you became gluten free?

How much better I feel every day! Running marathons. Climbing mountains. My body has healed in miraculous ways in the absence of the gluten toxin.

In ten years, a gluten free diet will be...

The gluten free diet will be the mainstay for most people, world-wide.

What is the best advice you received?

Test everyone!

What is the best way for people to connect with you?

Website: GlutenFreeRN.com

Instagram: @GlutenFreeRN

Email: Nadine@GlutenFreeRN

Best Gluten Free Bread Mixes

10th Annual Gluten-Free Awards:

1st Place Winner: King Arthur Gluten Free Flour Bread Mix

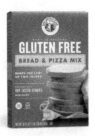

2nd Place Winner: gfJules Bread Mix

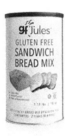

3rd Place Winner: Bob's Red Mill Gluten Free Hearty Whole Grain Bread Mix

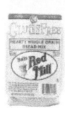

Other Great Products:

Pamela's Products Gluten-free Bread Mix

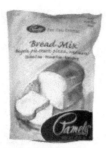

Simple Mills Almond Flour Mix, Artisan Bread

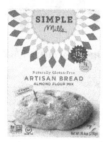

Chebe Gluten Free Original Cheese Bread Mix

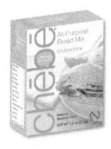

CELIAC SURVEY

We polled over 400 people with celiac disease
with the intent to make you feel not so alone.

Do you have anxiety when
eating out on a
gluten free diet?

77% Yes

23% No

Presented by The 2020 Gluten Free Buyers Guide

YOU'RE NOT ALONE

Best Gluten Free Breakfast On-The-Go

10th Annual Gluten-Free Awards:

1st Place Winner: KIND Protein Bars, White Chocolate Cinnamon Almond, Gluten Free

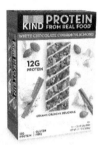

2nd Place Winner: Bobo's Strawberry Toaster Pastry

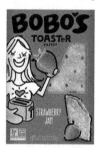

3rd Place Winner: Enjoy Life Foods Chocolate Chip Banana Breakfast Ovals

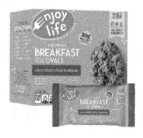

Other Great Products:

Mikey's Egg, Ham and Cheese Pocket

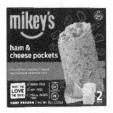

Bakery On Main Oats & Happiness Oatmeal Cups

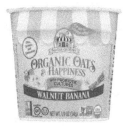

MadeGood Foods Apple Cinnamon Granola Bars

GF Harvest GoPack Single Serve Oatmeal Pack - Maple & Brown Sugar

Sweet PotaTOASTS, from the creators of CAULIPOWER - Roasted Sweet Potato Slices

Modern Oats Premium Organic Oatmeal Cups Apple Cinnamon Ginger

Lark Ellen Farm Grain Free Granola Bites, Vanilla Cinnamon

Meet Erin Smith

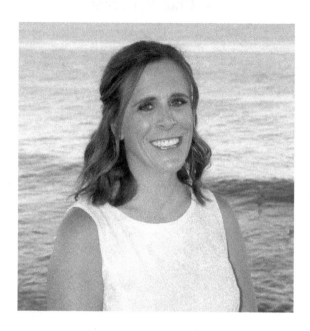

How long have you been gluten free?

I have been gluten-free since my celiac disease diagnosis way back in 1981!

Do you have any other dietary restrictions?

I have a shellfish allergy.

What has been your biggest challenge thus far?

As a kid growing up with celiac disease in the 1980s and '90s, it was really hard to find gluten-free food. Most people never heard of it and many supermarkets and restaurants had no gluten-free options. My biggest challenge today is getting people to take my celiac disease and need for gluten-free food seriously. I am not eating this way to be trendy. I am eating gluten-free because it is medically necessary.

Where is your favorite place to eat?

Italy! There are so many surprising and delicious gluten-free options in the land of pizza and pasta. Italians take gluten-free food very seriously.

Do you have any gluten related pet peeves?

I am really bothered by people who eat gluten-free by choice but then will order a gluten-filled beer or dessert. This makes it so much harder for those of us with celiac disease to be taken seriously.

Do you have any relatives are close friends that are gluten free?

Yes! My sister has celiac disease and at least one first cousin has been formally diagnosed. I suspect a few other family members also have celiac but have not been properly tested.

Do you have a gluten horror story?

I have too many from growing up with celiac disease when people didn't even know the words gluten-free.

I think my worst most recent "glutening" was on a trip to France and Germany. As soon as my plane landed in Berlin, I was running to be sick in the bathroom. I suspect something marked gluten-free in France wasn't really and it made me sick.

What has been the biggest change since you became gluten free?

There are SO many more options today than there were when I was diagnosed with celiac disease in the 1980s. My mom used to mail order food for me from across the country. Remember, this was way before the Internet was invented. Being able to walk into a grocery store and seeing several gluten-free products today was unimaginable back then.

In ten years, a gluten free diet will be...

medically necessary and hopefully taken much more seriously.

What is the best advice you received?

Growing up with celiac, my parents never treated me any differently from my sister who was not yet diagnosed except for my food. I always lived a "normal" life going to school, sleepaway camp, and traveling around the world. They instilled in me to never let celiac disease stop me from living my life.

What is the best way for people to connect with you?

My website is www.glutenfreeglobetrotter.com.

I am also on Twitter, Facebook, and Instagram @glutenfreeglobetrotter

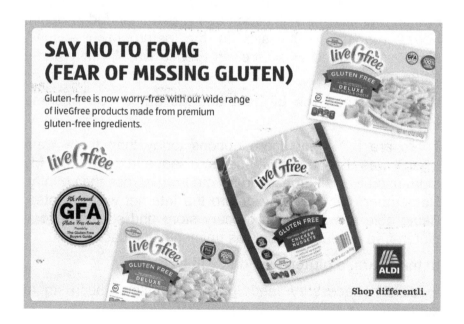

Best Gluten Free Brownie Mix

10th Annual Gluten-Free Awards:

1st Place Winner: Krusteaz Gluten Free Double Chocolate Brownie Mix

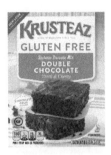

2nd Place Winner: King Arthur Flour Gluten Free Brownie Mix

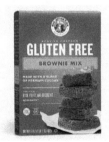

3rd Place Winner: Trader Joe's Gluten Free Chocolate Chip Brownie Mix

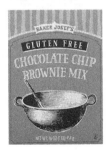

Other Great Products:

Pamela's Products Gluten Free Chocolate Brownie Mix

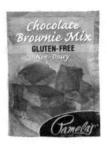

Glutino Brownie Mix

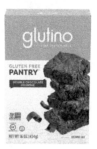

Enjoy Life Brownie Mix

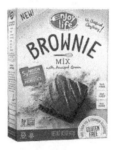

Gluten-Free Prairie Deep Dark Chocolate Brownie Mix

Best Gluten Free Buns

10th Annual Gluten-Free Awards:

1st Place Winner: Schar's Gluten Free Ciabatta Rolls

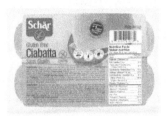

2nd Place Winner: Udi's Gluten Free Classic Hamburger Buns

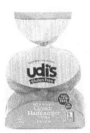

3rd Place Winner: Canyon Bakehouse Hamburger Buns

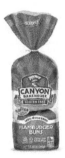

Other Great Products:

Three Bakers' Whole Grain Hamburger Buns

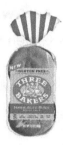

Smart Bun - Gluten Free, Zero carbs of sugar, sesame, Hamburger Buns

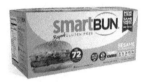

New Cascadia Traditional Gluten Free Hamburger Buns

CELIAC SURVEY

We polled over 400 people with celiac disease
with the intent to make you feel not so alone.

Do you like to eat out or at home?

84% Home

26% Out

Presented by The 2020 Gluten Free Buyers Guide

YOU'RE NOT ALONE

Meet Melinda Arcara

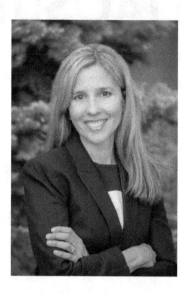

How long have you been gluten free?

11 years - WOW!

Do you have any other dietary restrictions?

Dairy Free and Gluten-Free

What has been your biggest challenge thus far?

I miss the spontaneity of just popping into a restaurant or cafe and meeting up with a group of friends for a drink. Because I like to call ahead to restaurants and be familiar where I eat, I don't accept as many invitations to go out with friends as I used to. I know other gluten intolerant sufferers feel the same way. The invites to go out may come, but the fear of not knowing what to eat, or accidental gluten exposure, prevents sufferers from accepting invitations. I am getting better at not waiting for invitations, but rather being the organizer and bringing friends together where everyone will enjoy and is gluten-free friendly.

Where is your favorite place to eat?

My husband and I love to golf and be outside, so we decided to seek out a place to play that would accommodate our special diet requirements. We interviewed kitchen staff at several country clubs in our region, but French Creek Country Club created a comfort level that we immediately felt. The club grows their own produce and herbs and even has their own honey hives on site. They even source local and seasonal ingredients from around the area, which we love. My favorite thing is to walk into the dining room and served a warm gluten-free roll with olive oil without even asking for it. What a simple thing to make me feel that the staff knows me personally and is aware of my gluten-free and dairy-free needs.

Do you have any gluten related pet peeves?

The one thing that really drives me crazy is when I introduce myself and my book to someone and they immediately try to discredit my credentials. No, I am not a registered dietitian, nor do I claim to be one. But, that doesn't mean that I don't know what I am talking about when it comes to eating gluten-free. I pride myself in being able to give newly diagnosed Celiac an Gluten-Intolerant sufferers practical advice and information. I have been eating a special diet for eleven years and have tried hundreds of products and supplements from all over the world. My goal has been to help newly diagnosed sufferers and supporters adhere to a gluten-free diet more easily than I did. Most people I have met after meeting with an RD are still left with the question of "Where do I start?". That's where my 3 Steps to Gluten-Free Living really helps people practically implement a new way of eating in their homes. From my own experience, people who do my 3 Step approach, in the order from elimination of gluten, to transitioning emotionally from foods and finally knowing what food substitutions are available saves patients time and money and helps them stay 100% gluten-free for life.

Do you have any relatives are close friends that are gluten free?

My sister Sue has been my gluten-free guru for the last 11 years. She was diagnosed with a gluten and dairy intolerance before me and really got me on my gluten-free journey. My sister, my husband (who is Celiac) and I travel all over the world together. He love planning our vacations together around our special eating requirements. It's so much more relaxing and enjoyable to be on vacation with family that has to eat the same way so you don't feel like anyone is being inconvenienced. Our favorite vacation spots have been Hawaii, Aruba and Palm Springs, CA.

Do you have a gluten horror story?

It's so much easier now to eat gluten-free than 11 years ago. When I first went gluten-free, I remember going into Panera Bread (WHAT WAS I THINKING) and asking for a soup with no croutons, thinking that was being careful enough. I put my spoon into my bowl and pulled out a crouton that had been saturated in the broth. I remember going out to my car and crying while my friends and family sat in the restaurant eating. I didn't want to ruin the meal for everyone else and felt so alone anticipating the affects of what that crouton would bring. I'm much wiser now and wouldn't hesitate to bring my own food into a restaurant to prevent being accidentally glutened.

What has been the biggest change since you became gluten free?

I love helping other people on their gluten-free journey. So many friends and family members that may not have been understanding of my gluten-free needs are now coming to me for advice about their own health journey or even a family members diagnosis. I love that more and more people are looking at food ingredients as a possible source for the symptoms. Food is medicine and it could be other peoples poison, so why not try a diet change to eliminate inflammation or pain?

In ten years, a gluten free diet will be...

Keeping balance with prepackaged gluten-free foods and naturally gluten-free foods. If you eat a diet that consists of 100% factory processed foods, you will gain weight and feel worse than before you went gluten-free. But, if you keep balance and eat foods grown in the sun, than the immune system will be stronger. No one wants to make a cracker or cereal, but why not add some fresh fruit or use local organic dairy items along with store bought items to make them a little healthier.

What is the best advice you received?

My brother Mark told me, "It's not how many books you sell, its how many people you have helped." Those words took the pressure off me with regards to how many books I sell on Amazon. If I sell one book to someone that is newly diagnosed, and helps them on their gluten-free journey, than that makes it worth all the while.

What is the best way for people to connect with you?

I know social media gets a lot of criticism, but I have helped so many people using Instagram (@glutenfreebebe) and Facebook. I love that people can send messages on these platforms and even make comments on pictures and articles. I read all the comments I receive and really try hard to connect with people, even if it's just a thumbs up or a smiling emoji. I really do care and want my followers to feel that.

Best Gluten Free Cake Mix

10th Annual Gluten-Free Awards:

1st Place Winner: Betty Crocker Gluten Free Yellow Cake Mix

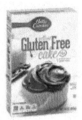

2nd Place Winner: King Arthur's Gluten Free Chocolate Cake Mix

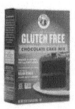

3rd Place Winner: King Arthur's Gluten Free Yellow Cake Mix

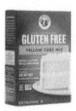

Other Great Products:

Pamela's Products Gluten Free Cake Mix, Classic Vanilla

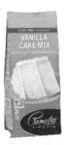

Better Batter Gluten Free Chocolate Cake Mix

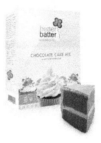

Cup4Cup Yellow Cake Mix

The Really Great Food Company Gluten Free Coffee Crumb Cake Mix

KNOW Foods - KNOW Better Muffin & Cake Mix

Best Gluten Free Candy

10th Annual Gluten-Free Awards:

1st Place Winner: Enjoy Life Chocolate Bar - Ricemilk Crunch

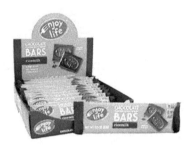

2nd Place Winner: Justin's Mini White Chocolate Peanut Butter Cups

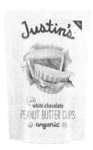

3rd Place Winner: Yum Earth Gummy Bears

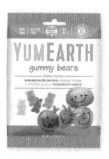

Other Great Products:

Jelly Belly Candy Corn

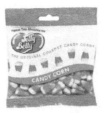

Undercover Quinoa- Dark Chocolate + Sea Salt

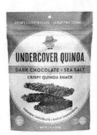

JJ's Sweets Sea Salt Chocolate-Covered Cocomels

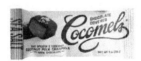

Gimbal's Scottie Dogs Strawberry Licorice

Honey Mama's Nibs & Coffee Cocoa Bar

Meet Carrie Veatch

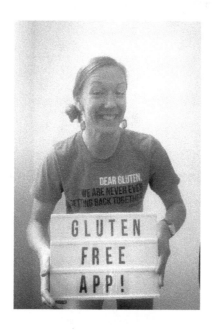

How long have you been gluten free?

8 years

Do you have any other dietary restrictions?

no

What has been your biggest challenge thus far?

I currently live and travel abroad so it is not always the easiest in the part of the world I am in (Asia). But it is getting easier and there are even many 100% gluten free spots popping up in Asia which are all included in my free dedicated gluten free app!

Where is your favorite place to eat?

So hard to choose! I've been in Asia for two years now and Bali was such a mecca for gluten free eating! Made's Banana Flour and Zest were absolutely incredible! In Denver (which is "home" for me) Quiero Arepas is one of my absolute favorites for arepas and Holidaily for beer!

Do you have any gluten related pet peeves?

Not really. I generally take most things that could be frustrating as an opportunity to educate others that might not understand!

Do you have any relatives are close friends that are gluten free?

I have lots of friends that are gluten free and even more all over the world since I've started my gluten free business!

Do you have a gluten horror story?

I definitely had to switch a flight once because I got glutened so badly I couldn't stay off the toilet so there was no way I would be able to fly... not sure if that's what you're going for :)

What has been the biggest change since you became gluten free?

My mental health. I struggled for so many years with depression and emotional volatility and once I healed my gut by going gluten free, everything changed! I truly have never been happier or healthier and am so grateful!

In ten years, a gluten free diet will be...

even more mainstream and so much simpler to navigate!

What is the best advice you received?

Eat foods that are naturally gluten free, i.e. shop the perimeter of the grocery store. And always be prepared! Definitely always lived this advice prior to my diagnosis with almost always having snacks on me, but now I simply travel with all the gluten free snacks!

What is the best way for people to connect with you?

Instagram   @forglutensake

Best Gluten Free Children's Book

10th Annual Gluten-Free Awards:

1st Place Winner: Eat Like a Dinosaur: Recipe & Guidebook for Gluten-free Kids by Paleo Parents and Elana Amsterdam

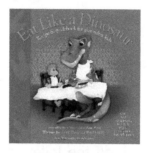

2nd Place Winner: Aidan the Wonder Kid Who Could Not Be Stopped: A Food Allergy and Intolerance Story by Dan Carsten and Colleen Brunetti

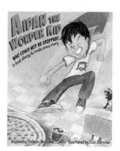

3rd Place Winner: Wheat-Free, Gluten-Free Cookbook for Kids and Busy Adults by Connie Sarros

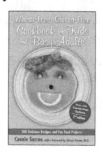

Other Great Products:

The GF Kid: A Celiac Disease Survival Guide by Melissa London and Eric Glickman

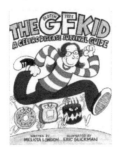

Adam's Gluten Free Surprise: Helping Others Understand Gluten Free by Debbie Simpson

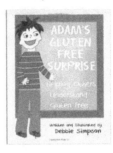

Eating Gluten-Free with Emily: A Story for Children with Celiac Disease by Bonnie J. Kruszka and Richard S. Cihlar

Gordy and the Magic Diet by Kim Diersen (Author), April Runge (Author), Carrie Hartman (Illustrator)

The Gluten Glitch by Stasie John and Kevin Cannon

CELIAC SURVEY

We polled over 400 people with celiac disease
with the intent to make you feel not so alone.

Opinion: How long will it take before they find a cure for Celiac Disease?

Average: 39 More Years

Presented by The 2020 Gluten Free Buyers Guide

YOU'RE NOT ALONE

Best Gluten Free Chips

10th Annual Gluten-Free Awards:

1st Place Winner: Cape Cod Waffle Cut Chips

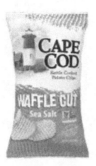

2nd Place Winner: UTZ - Ripple Potato Chips

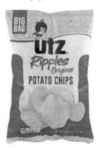

3rd Place Winner: Late July Snacks - Organic Multigrain Tortilla Chips Gluten Free Sea Salt By The Seashore

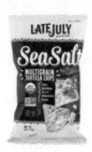

Other Great Products:

POPCORNERS Carnival Kettle, Popped Corn Chips, Gluten Free, Non-GMO

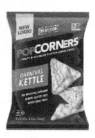

ALDI - liveGfree Gluten Free Sweet Chili Brown Rice Crisps

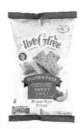

Enjoy Life Foods Sea Salt Lentil Chips

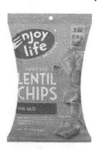

Way Better Snacks Sprouted Gluten Free Tortilla Chips Unbeatable Blues

Beanfields Bean and Rice Chips - Nacho

Meet Hayley Johnston

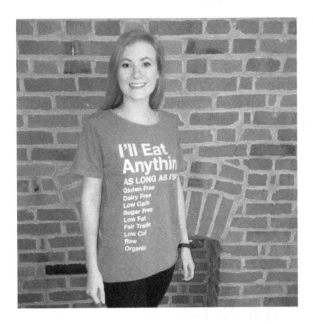

How long have you been gluten free?

Since 2013 (6 years)

Do you have any other dietary restrictions?

Food Intolerances to mushrooms, pineapple, and lettuce.

What has been your biggest challenge thus far?

Maintaining my social life.

Where is your favorite place to eat?

The Corner Pub and Grill in Valley Park, MO

Do you have any gluten related pet peeves?

When people ask if I can eat potatoes. I don't know why but it drives me nuts! But is a great opportunity for some gluten education.

Do you have any relatives are close friends that are gluten free?

My aunt is celiac and my cousin is gluten intolerant.

Do you have a gluten horror story?

I once got glutened at an out of town wedding which was definitely not fun. I don't have a horror story that I can think of but that could be because I blocked it out of my memory.

What has been the biggest change since you became gluten free?

Having Celiac Disease means always having to stand up for yourself and be your own advocate and that has carried over into all parts of my life, not just about what I consume.

In ten years, a gluten free diet will be...

Hopefully not necessary because we will have a cure ;)

What is the best advice you received?

To advocate for myself because no one else knows me as well as I do.

What is the best way for people to connect with you?

On my instagram and @sociableceliac

Best Gluten Free Cold Cereal

10th Annual Gluten-Free Awards:

1st Place Winner: Cinnamon Rice Chex

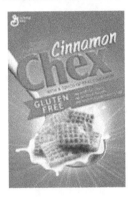

2nd Place Winner: Post Cocoa Pebbles

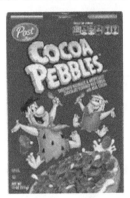

3rd Place Winner: Nature's Path Organic Mesa Sunrise Cereal

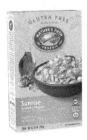

Other Great Products:

Bakery On Main Gluten Free Granola

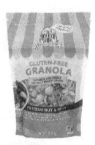

purely elizabeth Probiotic Gluten Free Granola, Chocolate Sea Salt

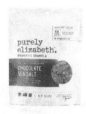

Bakery On Main Dark Chocolate Sea Salt Bunches of Crunches GrainOLA

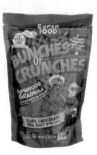

Love Grown Comet Crispies Cereal

Autumn's Gold Maple Grain Free Granola

Best Gluten Free Accommodating Colleges

10th Annual Gluten-Free Awards:

1st Place Winner: UNIVERSITY OF NOTRE DAME

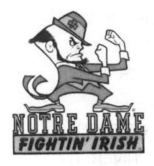

2nd Place Winner: MICHIGAN STATE

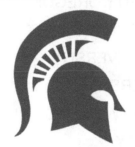

3rd Place Winner: UNIVERSITY OF COLORADO: BOULDER

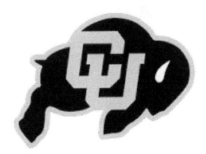

Other Great Schools:

UNIVERSITY OF TENNESSEE

UNIVERSITY OF CALIFORNIA, LOS ANGELES

UNIVERSITY OF ARIZONA

YALE UNIVERSITY

NC STATE UNIVERSITY

UNIV OF OREGON

IOWA STATE UNIVERSITY

ITHACA COLLEGE

KENT STATE UNIVERSITY

OREGON STATE UNIVERSITY

PACIFIC UNIVERSITY OREGON

UNIVERSITY OF CONNECTICUT

GEORGETOWN UNIVERSITY

COLUMBIA UNIVERSITY

UNIVERSITY OF NEW HAMPSHIRE

CLARK UNIVERSITY

TOWSON UNIVERSITY

CARLETON COLLEGE

CELIAC SURVEY

We polled over 400 people with celiac disease with the intent to make you feel not so alone.

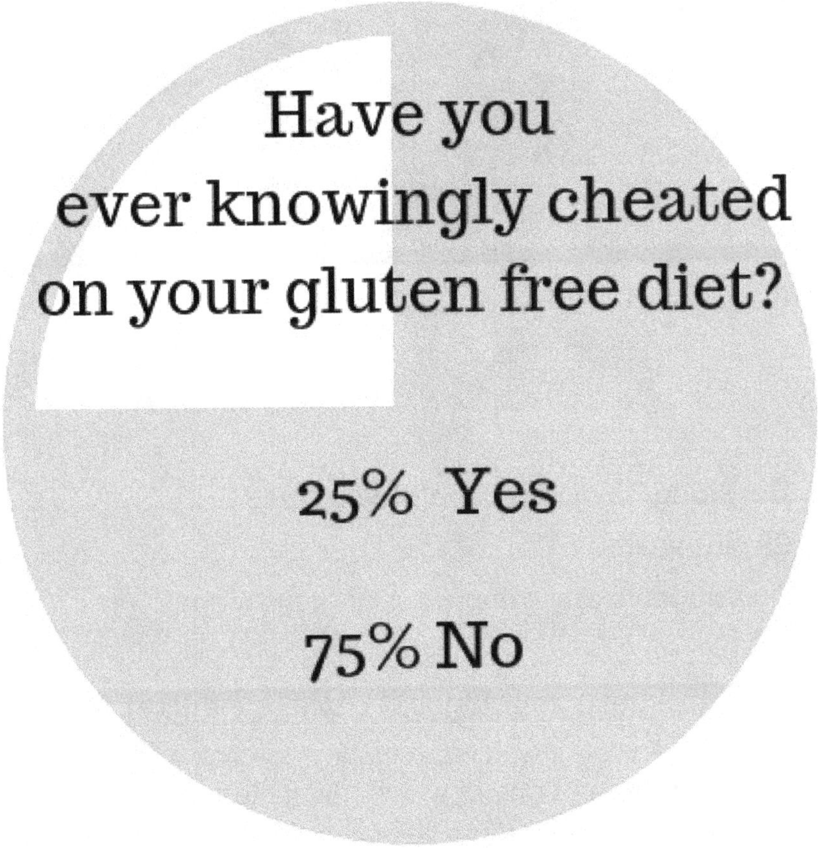

Have you
ever knowingly cheated
on your gluten free diet?
25% Yes
75% No

Presented by The 2020 Gluten Free Buyers Guide

YOU'RE NOT ALONE

Meet Carol Kicinski

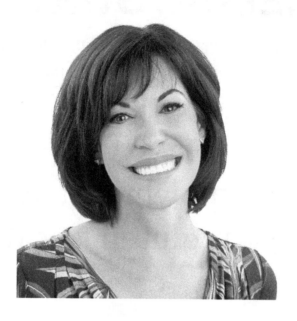

How long have you been gluten free?

25 plus years

Do you have any other dietary restrictions?

No

What has been your biggest challenge thus far?

In the beginning it was learning how to cook and eat without all my favorites - none of which had gluten-free replacements at the time. Now, it is second nature to me. I will say however, I find catered events challenging.

Where is your favorite place to eat?

Home! But I have found a lot of local restaurants that do gluten free really well. Senza Gluten in NYC is a big favorite!

Do you have any gluten related pet peeves?

When people assume that a little gluten is ok.

Do you have any relatives are close friends that are gluten free?

Yes - most of my family.

Do you have a gluten horror story?

Traveling through China was a nightmare. I loved the country but it was by far the most difficult place for me to eat. I came home after several weeks gluten poisoned!

What has been the biggest change since you became gluten free?

I am healthier now, 25 years later, than I was before. I suffered from weekly migraines. Thankfully going gluten free handled that.

In ten years, a gluten free diet will be...

So common place!

What is the best advice you received?

Don't cheat. Ever!

What is the best way for people to connect with you?

Through my website - simplygluten-free.com

Best Gluten Free Comfort Food

10th Annual Gluten-Free Awards:

1st Place Winner: Goodie Girl Cookies - Mint Cookies

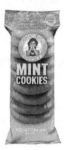

2nd Place Winner: Annie's Gluten Free Rice Pasta & Cheddar

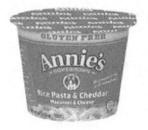

3rd Place Winner: CAULIPOWER Cauliflower Pizza

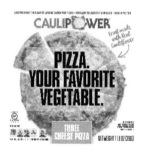

Other Great Products:

Amy's Gluten Free Frozen Mac and Cheese

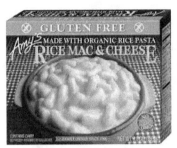

ALDI - liveGfree Gluten Free Stuffed Sandwiches: Ham & Cheese

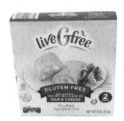

CAULIPOWER Chicken Tenders

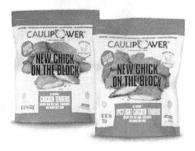

Gratify - Cinnamon Baked Bites

Lightlife Plant-Based Burger

Best Gluten Free Cookbooks

10th Annual Gluten-Free Awards:

1st Place Winner: Free for All Cooking: 150 Easy Gluten-Free, Allergy-Friendly Recipes the Whole Family Can Enjoy by Jules E. Dowler Shepard

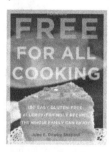

2nd Place Winner : Danielle Walker's Eat What You Love: Everyday Comfort Food You Crave; Gluten-Free, Dairy-Free, and Paleo Recipes: A Cookbook by Danielle Walker

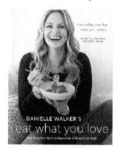

3rd Place Winner: The Easy Gluten-Free Cookbook: Fast and Fuss-Free Recipes for Busy People on a Gluten-Free Diet by Lindsay Garza

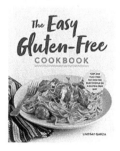

Other Great Products:

The Cake Mix Doctor Bakes Gluten-Free by Anne Byrn

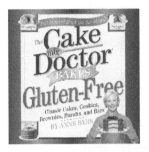

The Whole30: The 30-Day Guide to Total Health and Food Freedom by Hartwig Urban, Melissa and Dallas Hartwig

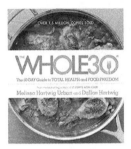

The Gluten-Free Quick Breads Cookbook: 75 Easy Homemade Loaves in Half the Time by Sharon Lachendro

Cook Once, Eat All Week: 26 Weeks of Gluten-Free, Affordable Meal Prep to Preserve Your Time & Sanity by Cassy Joy Garcia

Eat Happy: Gluten Free, Grain Free, Low Carb Recipes For A Joyful Life by Anna Vocino

Practical Paleo, 2nd Edition (Updated and Expanded): A Customized Approach to Health and a Whole-Foods Lifestyle by Diane Sanfilippo and Bill Staley

Hassle Free, Gluten Free by Jane Devonshire

Gluten Free Way: Thrive on Your Gluten Free Journey by Julianne Morrison

DID YOU KNOW?

CELIAC DISEASE: INCREASED TO 3% IN US (NOT 1% AS CONSISTENTLY REPORTED)

Quoted from:
17th International Celiac Disease
Symposium in New Delhi, India

Meet Jessica Hanson

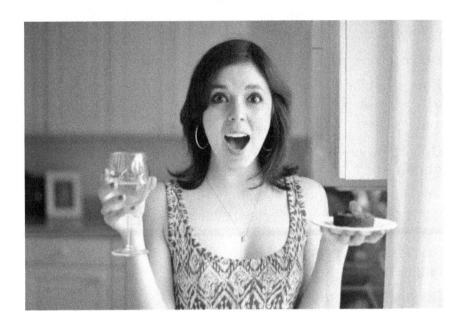

How long have you been gluten free?

I have been strictly gluten free since my celiac disease diagnosis in 2011.

Do you have any other dietary restrictions?

Soy is not my friend, though I can tolerate limited quantities every so often.

What has been your biggest challenge thus far?

I ended a long-term relationship because my now-ex bullied me about celiac disease. It was an emotionally difficult time, but it was perhaps the best decision I've ever made. A month after breaking it off I met my now-husband who is a dream. From the beginning he was understanding, protective and thoughtful. He was the one who convinced me to start a blog, and he continues to show overwhelming support and enthusiasm for my advocacy.

Where is your favorite place to eat?

My newest favorite place to eat is Mama Eat in Rome! My husband and I went there three or four times during our honeymoon, and we can't wait to go back!

Do you have any gluten related pet peeves?

How much time do you have? Restaurants advertising foods that are heavily contaminated as "gluten free" really upsets me. It's much more than a pet peeve.

Do you have any relatives are close friends that are gluten free?

Yes, I have several family members who are gluten free, and many of my close friends have celiac. I'm fortunate to have met hundreds of gluten free individuals through my blog and the NYC Celiac Disease Meetup Group, of which I am an organizer.

Do you have a gluten horror story?

Yes, and it still gives me nightmares. It's a long story, but what it boils down to is it's difficult to know who you can trust.

What has been the biggest change since you became gluten free?

My whole life changed. I've always been a big believer of sticking up for what you believe in, but when I was diagnosed I didn't know that in a few years I would be organizing events for the largest gluten free Meetup group in the world or sitting in my senator's office talking about the importance of the Gluten in Medications Disclosure Act. I'm incredibly passionate about this community and have met so many wonderful people. I'm so honored to be an advocate.

In ten years, a gluten free diet will be...

No longer a fad (I hope!)

What is the best advice you received?

Never apologize for what you need.

What is the best way for people to connect with you?

Through my blog www.TastyMeditation.com and through the NYC Celiac Disease Meetup Group (www.meetup.com/celiac)! I'm also on Instagram, twitter and Facebook as @TastyMeditation. I'm always happy to chat!

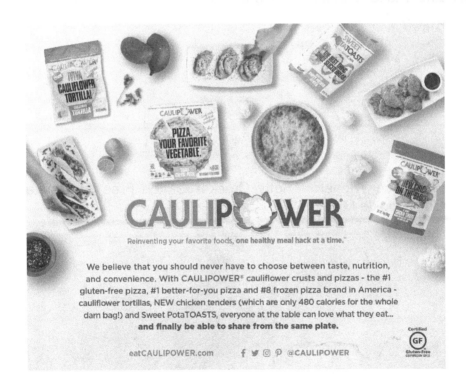

Best Gluten Free Cookie Mixes

10th Annual Gluten-Free Awards:

1st Place Winner: gfJules Cookie Mix

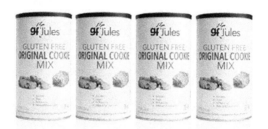

2nd Place Winner: Krusteaz Gluten Free Chocolate Chip Cookie Mix

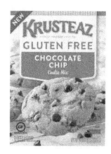

3rd Place Winner: Betty Crocker Gluten Free Chocolate Chip Cookie Mix

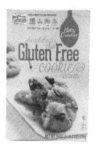

Other Great Products:

Pamela's Products Gluten Free Chocolate Chunk Cookie Mix

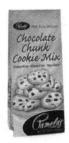

Simple Mills Chocolate Chip Cookie Mix

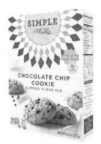

Hodgson Mill Gluten Free Cookie Mix

Meli's Monster Gluten Free Cookies (Original)

XO Baking Gourmet Sugar Cookie Mix

123 Gluten Free Lindsay's Lipsmackin' Roll-Out & Cut Sugar Cookies

Bella Gluten-Free Chocolate Chip Cookie Mix

CELIAC SURVEY

We polled over 400 people with celiac disease with the intent to make you feel not so alone.

After consuming gluten, do you have symptoms?

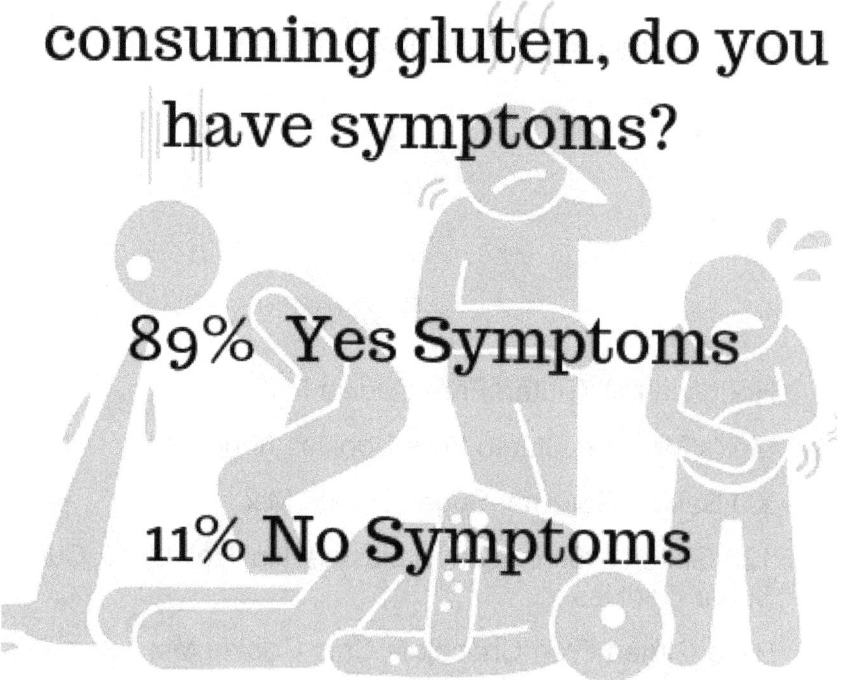

89% Yes Symptoms

11% No Symptoms

Presented by The 2020 Gluten Free Buyers Guide

YOU'RE NOT ALONE

Best Gluten Free Cookies

10th Annual Gluten-Free Awards:

1st Place Winner: Goodie Girl Gluten Free Cookies - Mint Cookies

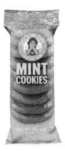

2nd Place Winner: Tate's Gluten Free Chocolate Chip Cookies

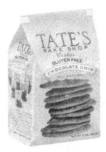

3rd Place Winner: Enjoy Life Foods Double Chocolate Brownie Soft Baked Cookies

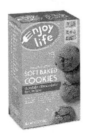

Other Great Products:

Pamela's Products Chunky Chocolate Chip Cookies

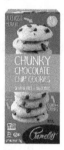

Glutino Gluten Free Wafer Cookies – Lemon

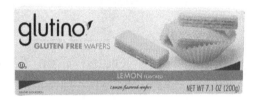

Schär: Chocolate Dipped Cookies

Simple Mills Crunchy Gluten Free Cookies - Double Chocolate

Cybele's Free-to-Eat Chocolate Chip Vegan & Gluten Free Cookies

Steve & Andy's Soft Baked Vegan Oatmeal Coconut Cookie

Steve & Andy's Crispy Chocolate Chip Cookies

Meet Dr. Tom O'Bryan

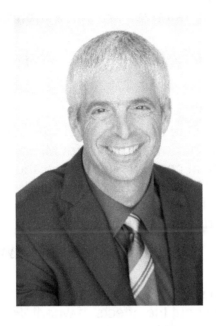

How long have you been gluten free?

since 1979 when we learned sensitivity to wheat was inhibiting our ability to achieve pregnancy

Do you have any other dietary restrictions?

Dairy

What has been your biggest challenge thus far?

releasing the 'comfort food' cravings for wheat when life is accumulating more stress than my threshold can handle without cravings

Where is your favorite place to eat?

Good On Ya, Encinitas, California

Do you have any gluten related pet peeves?

the refusal of our Manufacturers to produce true GF foods. and the now-proven fact that 50.8% of all GF pastas and

53.2% of all GF pizzas in restaurants are not GF!
American Journal of Gastroenterology 2019;00:1–6

Do you have any relatives are close friends that are gluten free?

a few. and, gratefully, tens of thousands of patients and Readers

Do you have a gluten horror story?

There are many. One that stands out was the young man who proposed to his love, a Resident MD, and had a wheelchair there in case she fainted, as she was the 'canary in the coal mine' with any wheat exposure, she would faint. He was not GF, but if he ate wheat within 24 hours of kissing her, she would have a reaction and faint.

What has been the biggest change since you became gluten free?

It's wonderful to see the world becoming more knowledgeable about the effects of wheat. Research is being published now all over the world about the dangers of wheat, with or without Celiac Disease. Our Health Practitioners are learning more all the time about the many manifestations of Wheat Related Disorders outside the gut.

In ten years, a gluten free diet will be...

the norm. As the science becomes more accepted that EVERY HUMAN gets transient Intestinal Permeability every time they're exposed to wheat, it will become more understood that any and every chronic health condition may be fueled by a sensitivity to wheat.   Journal of the American Medical Association, August 15, 2017 Volume 318, Number 7

What is the best advice you received?

Look with eyes that see, listen with ears that hear

What is the best way for people to connect with you?

www.theDr.com

Best Gluten Free Cornbread Mix

10th Annual Gluten-Free Awards:

1st Place Winner: Krusteaz Gluten Free Cornbread Mix

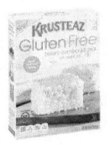

2nd Place Winner: Bob's Red Mill Gluten Free Cornbread Mix

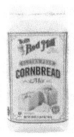

3rd Place Winner: gfJules Cornbread Mix

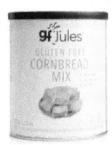

Other Great Products:

King Arthur Flour, Cornbread + Muffin Mix, Gluten Free

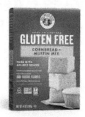

Pamela's Gluten Free Cornbread Mix

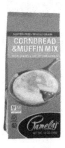

Glutino Cornbread Mix

Good Dee's Corn Bread Baking Mix - Grain Free, Sugar Free, Gluten Free, Wheat Free, and Low Carb

Really Great Food Company – Gluten Free Cornbread Muffin Mix

Best Gluten Free Cosmetic Brands

10th Annual Gluten-Free Awards:

1st Place Winner: tarte

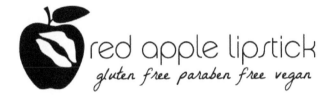

2nd Place Winner: Arbonne

℥ ARBONNE

3rd Place Winner: Red Apple Lipstick

red apple lipstick

gluten free paraben free vegan

Other Great Products:

Au Naturale

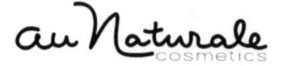

Afterglow

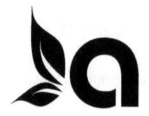

Kiss Freely

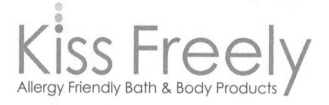

Gabriel Cosmetics

Lily Lolo

ILIA Beauty

CELIAC SURVEY

We polled over 400 people with celiac disease
with the intent to make you feel not so alone.

Do you have other family with Celiac Disease?

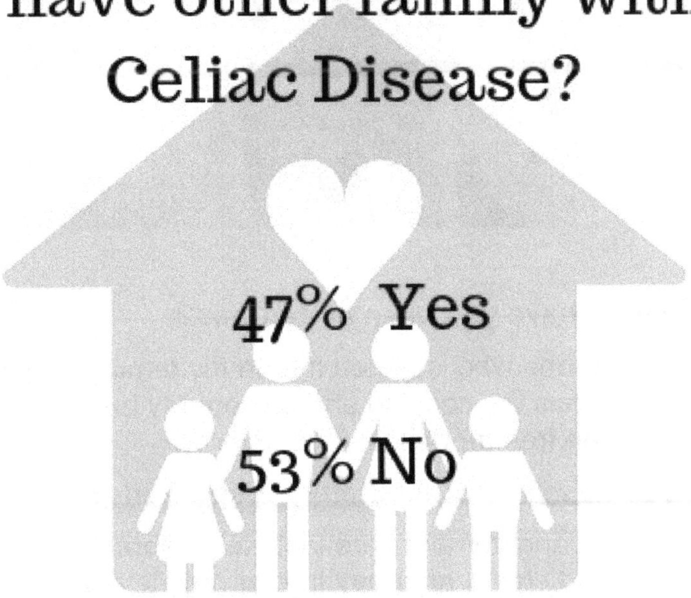

47% Yes

53% No

Presented by The 2020 Gluten Free Buyers Guide

YOU'RE NOT ALONE

Meet Sharon Lachendro

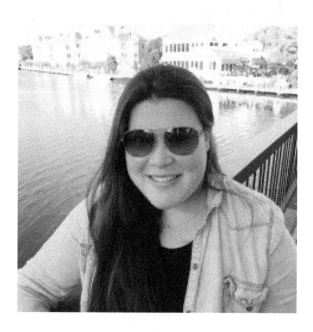

How long have you been gluten free?

I'm not the one who is gluten free in my family, I'm just the one who does the cooking and baking! My husband has been gluten free for almost 7 years now.

Do you have any other dietary restrictions?

My oldest daughter and I are lactose intolerant so many of the recipes I create are dairy free or have a dairy free option.

What has been your biggest challenge thus far?

Teaching myself to bake all over again was hard. It took a lot of trial and error and a lot of failed attempts. The effort was well worth it though.

Where is your favorite place to eat?

We don't eat out often but we love Red Robin when my husband wants a burger on a good bun! We also like Legal

Seafoods (Boston based). We also love Pizzetta in Mystic, CT.

Do you have any relatives are close friends that are gluten free?

My cousin's husband was just diagnosed with Celiac Disease this past year. My mom and my aunt have also been gluten free for several years - my mom has been gluten free for about 10 years.

What has been the biggest change since you became gluten free?

Creating gluten free baked goods that taste just as good, if not better than baked goods made with regular flour is a huge challenge. But I love every second of recipe testing and it's so rewarding when I finally nail a recipe.

In ten years, a gluten free diet will be...

I can't wait to see what's available in ten years. There are so many new products hitting shelves all the time. I'm hoping in ten years the options will be endless!

What is the best way for people to connect with you?

Instagram: whattheforkfoodblog Or in my Facebook group - Gluten Free Baking Club
https://www.facebook.com/groups/glutenfreebakingclub/

Best Gluten Free Crackers

10th Annual Gluten-Free Awards:

1st Place Winner: Schär Table Crackers

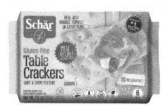

2nd Place Winner: Blue Diamond Almond Nut Thins Cracker Crisps, Hint of Sea Salt

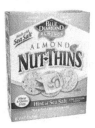

3rd Place Winner: Crunchmaster Gluten Free Protein Snack Crackers, Sea Salt

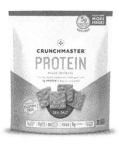

Other Great Products:

Mary's Gone Crackers Super Seed Everything

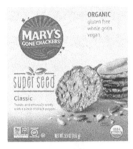

Mary's Gone Crackers Original

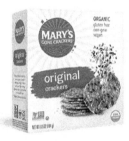

Three Bakers Real Cheddar Snackers

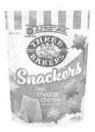

Mary's Gone Crackers REAL Thin Crackers Sea Salt

San-J Gluten Free Tamari Black Sesame Crackers

Jilz Gluten Free Tuscan Crackerz (Lemon and Herbs)

Best Gluten Free Donuts

10th Annual Gluten-Free Awards:

1st Place Winner: Katz Gluten Free, Glazed Donuts

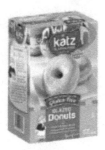

2nd Place Winner: Katz Gluten Free, Glazed Chocolate Donut Holes

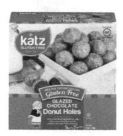

3rd Place Winner: Katz Gluten Free, Powdered Donut

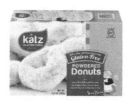

Other Great Products:

Kinnikinnick Gluten Free Vanilla Glazed Donut

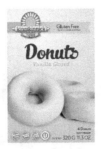

Kinnikinnick Gluten Free Maple Glazed Donut

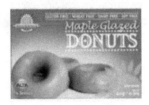

Ello Raw Organic Snacks Cinnamon Donut Bites

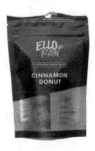

Meet Matt Hansen

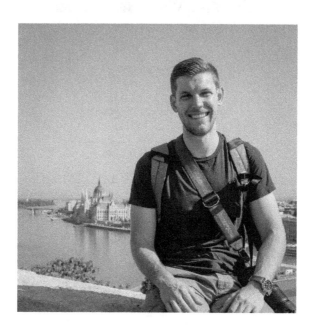

How long have you been gluten free?

I have been diagnosed with Celiac Disease for just over 10 years.

Do you have any other dietary restrictions?

Nope!

What has been your biggest challenge thus far?

The social side of having Celiac Disease is always going to be the biggest challenge for me. It basically comes down to not being able to be as spontaneous or flexible as I'd like to be.

It's the work events, social get-togethers ("Hey! Let's grab dinner after work!"), and even weddings that are hardest.

I have two strategies that I use to make it a little easier to have a social life with Celiac Disease.

First, I ALWAYS offer to plan things. Camping trips. Happy hours. Dinner parties. I'll offer to make a menu, pick a place, etc. Most of the time this works, but probably not for bigger group, friends that you aren't as close with, and work events. Which leads me to my second point.

Second, I don't hesitate to bring my own food or eat beforehand. For situations that I can't really control, like weddings or work events, I'll bring my own food. For things like dinner parties, I'll eat in advance, bring some snacks, and just enjoy some wine or cider and good company.

Where is your favorite place to eat?

It's definitely Ghostfish Brewing Company in Seattle. Not only are they a 100% gluten free restaurant, they also brew some of the best 100% gluten free beer around!

They hold a special place in my heart because they are the first 100% gluten free beer I ever tried that is actually good.

Back in 2012, there basically weren't any good 100% gluten free beer options on the market that I had found (brewed with gluten free grains, not gluten-reduced which I won't drink). Which was a bummer, because I like beer. So I learned to love cider and wine. But I still missed beer.

Enter Ghostfish.

I had been diagnosed for a few years and was living in Seattle. Since my diagnosis, I had found exactly zero good 100% gluten free beers. I vividly remember the first time I visited their taproom and trying two things. First, their Grapefruit IPA, which is still one of my favorite beers. Second, their fish and chips, which are 100% gluten free, and 100% delicious.

If you're visiting Seattle, Ghostfish is on the way into the city from the airport. It's always my first AND last stop on the way to or from the airport. And it probably should be yours too.

Pushkin's Bakery in Sacramento, California is close second. Their gluten free donuts on Sundays are to die for.

Do you have any gluten related pet peeves?

If you bake something for me, like cookies or a birthday cake, you're putting me in a really awkward position of having to say "thanks but no thanks."

I don't know what ingredients you used, what pans you cooked in, whether that wooden spoon you used has been used for regular cookies. The list goes on and on and on.

I always tell people not to cook for me, because 95% of the time it gets awkward.

Do you have any relatives are close friends that are gluten free?

None of my close friends eat gluten free. Unless they're with me. My friends are all super supportive, going as far as eating gluten free on our annual camping trip to make it easier for me.

My wife eats 99% gluten free because of me. Our house is basically 100% gluten free with the exception of one pan and one wooden spoon that she uses when she needs her regular pasta fix.

My immediate family has all been tested for Celiac Disease and none of them have it. That being said, whenever I'm in town, we all usually eat 100% gluten free to make everything easier.

Do you have a gluten horror story?

I don't really have any memorable horror stories that go "I ate X and then found out it had gluten in it, oh no!"

My biggest horror story happened early on in my gluten free travel journey. On an international flight, they forgot my gluten free meal. I ordered it. I even called to confirm it. They just straight up forgot it.

The flight attendants were super apologetic, but that didn't change the fact that I was stuck in a flying metal tube for 12 hours with only a few snack bars to get me through.

I was probably not the most pleasant person to be around for those 12 hours. I definitely had a case of the hangries.

I learned my lesson. Now, I always bring backup snacks on long flights. I still order the gluten free meal, but I'll also pack a sandwich, some crackers, nuts, protein bars, etc. Just to make sure I'm covered if I don't get fed on that flight.

Q9What has been the biggest change since you became gluten free?

Too many to count, most of them positive.

But the biggest change has to be that I have become a much better cook. Early on, it was a lot of chicken breast, brown rice, and barbecue sauce. Today? Can't find a restaurant that serves something I want to eat that is safe for Celiacs, like Indian food? Now I'll just make it myself. I LOVE my Instant Pot.

Food is still a big part of travel for me, and I'll gladly do hours of research to find the best & safest gluten free eats around the world. One of my favorite things to do is to try and recreate the foods I eat abroad in my kitchen at home.

I was so impressed by deliciousness of every single corn tortilla I ate in Mexico City (seriously, I didn't know a corn tortilla could be so good) that I ordered a tortilla press while I was still there so it was waiting for me when I got home. Now, I usually make my own tortillas when we're having tacos (spoiler: they're not even close to as good as the ones in Mexico City).

In ten years, a gluten free diet will be...

Better understood by the scientific community, and probably less trendy.

What is the best advice you received?

ABS. Always. Bring. Snacks. Especially when you're traveling and unsure if you'll be able to find safe gluten free food.   Nobody likes you when you're hangry.

What is the best way for people to connect with you?

You can check out my blog at WheatlessWanderlust.com. My mission is to inspire and empower people with Celiac Disease to have unforgettable gluten free travel experiences and start checking things off their bucket list. You'll find in-depth Celiac City Guides with the best things to do, see, and of course, eat in cities around the world like San Francisco, Rome, Paris, and even New Zealand.

You can also find me on Instagram where I'm @Wheatless_Wanderlust - follow along on my travels around the world with Celiac Disease.

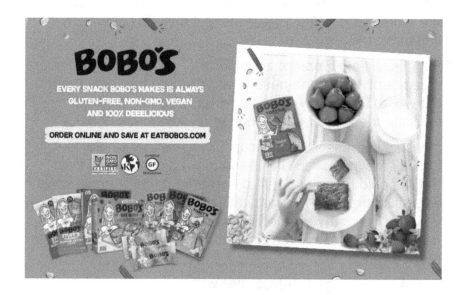

Best Gluten Free Expo and Events

10th Annual Gluten-Free Awards:

1st Place Winner: Living Free Expo (formerly Gluten & Allergen Free Wellness Events)

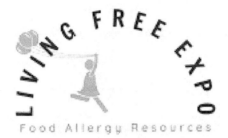

2nd Place Winner: The Nourished Festival (formerly GFAF Expo)

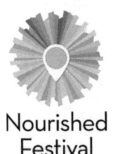

3rd Place Winner: Natural Expo West

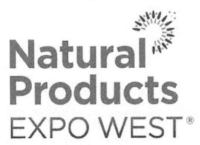

Other Great Gluten Free Expos:

CDF National Education & Gluten-Free Expo

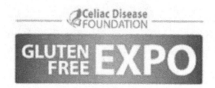

Natural Products Expo East

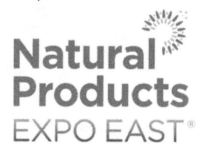

Central PA Gluten Free Expo

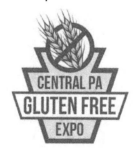

CELIAC SURVEY

We polled over 400 people with celiac disease with the intent to make you feel not so alone.

At work, are you the only one with Celiac Disease?

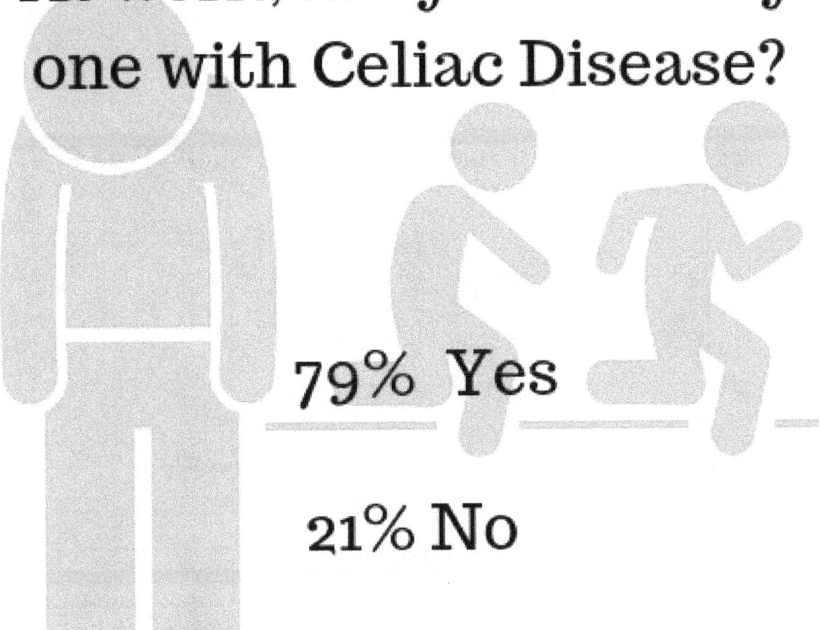

79% Yes

21% No

Presented by The 2020 Gluten Free Buyers Guide

YOU'RE NOT ALONE

Best Gluten Free Flours

10th Annual Gluten-Free Awards:

1st Place Winner: Bob's Red Mill Gluten Free 1-to-1 Baking Flour

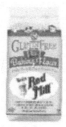

2nd Place Winner: gfJules All Purpose Gluten Free Flour

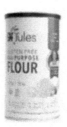

3rd Place Winner: King Arthur Gluten Free Flour

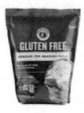

Other Great Products:

Cup 4 Cup™ Gluten Free Flour Blend

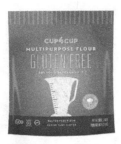

Otto's Naturals Cassava Flour

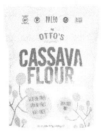

Enjoy Life All-Purpose Flour

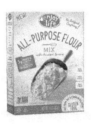

Nutiva Organic Coconut Flour

Domata Gluten Free Recipe Ready Flour

Gluten-Free Prairie Simply Wholesome All Purpose Flour Blend

Anthony's Organic Tiger Nut Flour

Meet Erica Dermer

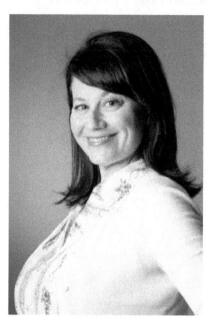

How long have you been gluten free?

I've been gluten free since 2009, with a few stints of gluten for proper testing and re-testing.

Do you have any other dietary restrictions?

Yes, I'm dairy-free, egg-free (baked okay), and beef-free

What has been your biggest challenge thus far?

While food has come a long way, restaurants are still the biggest challenge! Most don't understand the opportunities for cross-contact in the back of the house.

Where is your favorite place to eat?

I'm so lucky to travel a lot for work. My favorites city is Portland, Oregon. There are so many safe restaurants and bakeries!

Do you have any gluten related pet peeves?

I really dislike people who go gluten free for a weight-loss diet - still, even after all these years - it makes it harder for those of us on a medical diet to eat for a disease.

Do you have any relatives are close friends that are gluten free?

My partner goes gluten-free in the house so we can keep it strictly gluten free! I'm so thankful for that.

Do you have a gluten horror story?

I was out at a fancy restaurant with my friends and I ordered spatzle gluten-free, and after I was done eating it - I found out that the waiter didn't understand what I had asked, and that it was gluten-full!

What has been the biggest change since you became gluten free?

I've changed my entire life after being diagnosed. I wrote a book about celiac disease - something I would have never done before. Now, I speak openly about health problems, and that's something I never would have pictured for myself!

In ten years, a gluten free diet will be...

Even easier than now! Hopefully with some sort of pharmaceutical intervention to make it easier to dine out!

What is the best advice you received?

You're more than your disease.

What is the best way for people to connect with you?

Check me out on Instagram @CeliacandtheBeast or CeliacandtheBeast.com!

Best Gluten Free Frozen Foods

10th Annual Gluten-Free Awards:

1st Place Winner: Amy's Frozen Gluten Free Bean and Cheese Burritos

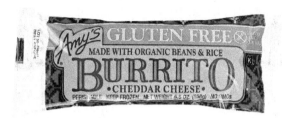

2nd Place Winner: Feel Good Foods Egg Rolls (veggie)

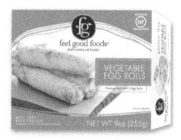

3rd Place Winner: CAULIPOWER Chicken Tenders

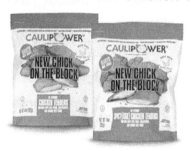

Other Great Products:

Feel Good Foods Potstickers (chicken)

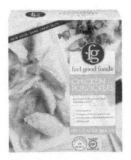

Mikey's Pepperoni Pizza Pockets

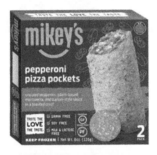

Feel Good Foods Empanadas (chicken)

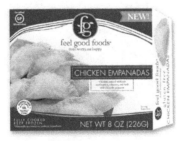

Feel Good Foods Taquitos (pinto bean & cheddar)

Feel Good Foods Snack Bites (3 cheese)

Swiss Rösti

Best Gluten Free Frozen Meals

10th Annual Gluten-Free Awards:

1st Place Winner: Amy's Rice Mac & Cheese, Gluten Free

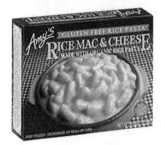

2nd Place Winner: Feel Good Foods Chicken Potstickers

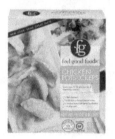

3rd Place Winner: ALDI - liveGfree Gluten Free Stuffed Sandwiches: Buffalo Chicken

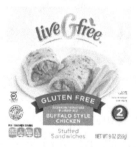

Other Great Products:

ALDI - liveGfree Gluten Free Stuffed Sandwiches: Spinach, Artichoke and Kale

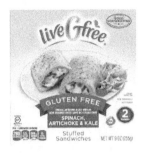

Saffron Road Lamb Saag with Basmati Rice

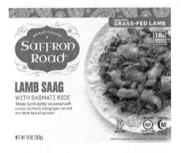

Mikey's Pepperoni Pizza Pockets

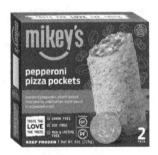

ALDI - liveGfree Gluten Free Stuffed Sandwiches: Southwest Veggie

Mikey's Cheese Pizza Pockets

CELIAC SURVEY

We polled over 400 people with celiac disease
with the intent to make you feel not so alone.

Do you drink gluten removed beer or stick to gluten free beers?

88% Gluten Free Only

5% Gluten Removed

7% Both

Presented by The 2020 Gluten Free Buyers Guide

YOU'RE NOT ALONE

Meet Jackie McEwan

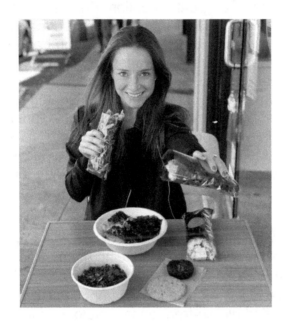

How long have you been gluten free?

7+ years

Do you have any other dietary restrictions?

Just gluten.

What has been your biggest challenge thus far?

My biggest challenge was when I found out that I had to follow a gluten-free diet. I was completely overwhelmed. I didn't even know what gluten was! I had to figure out what foods I could eat, what foods I had to avoid, and the nuances in between. I wished I had a go to guide to tell me all I needed to know about following a gluten-free diet. This manual did not yet exist so I did a ton of research and learned how to maneuver being gluten-free at restaurants and in my own kitchen.

In March 2014, I started to post about some of the gluten-free foods I was eating on Instagram. Surprisingly to me, my posts were met with great reception. People I had never met were asking me for more tips on gluten-free friendly eateries, products, and recipes, and I was more than happy to continue to make these discoveries. I was getting so many questions that I knew I needed to put all this information in one place rather than just Instagram. In September 2014, I taught myself how to make a website, and I launched glutenfreefollowme.com! I wish I had something like Gluten Free Follow Me to guide me through my new gluten-free diet seven years ago, but I'm glad I can be a guide for others now!

At the time, going gluten-free seemed like the worst thing ever. However, I'm grateful for it now. Knowledge is power, and I'm healthier because of it. Going gluten-free lead me to start Gluten Free Follow Me. If I hadn't become gluten-free, I would probably still be working in finance in New York City. My quest to find gluten-free foods developed into a full-time passion, and I couldn't be happier with how it all turned out!

Where is your favorite place to eat?

I have many favorites! A few of my faves are: - Beaming (LA) - Posh Pop Bakeshop (NYC) - Little Beet Table (NYC + CT + Chicago) - Vibe Organic Kitchen (Newport Beach)

Do you have any gluten related pet peeves?

When someone says that they could never give up gluten. When you have to, yes you can! And honestly, it's not that hard, especially nowadays. There are so many amazing options.

Do you have any relatives are close friends that are gluten free?

Yes! I have many friends that are also gluten-free. This number has gone up in the last few years.

Do you have a gluten horror story?

Back when I was working in NYC, I went out to lunch at a restaurant that is now closed. I told the hostess, manager, and waitress that I was gluten-free. They went through the menu with me and told me which options were safe for me to eat. I ended up ordering the nachos as an appetizer. I had just taken my first bite of the nachos when the manager ran over to tell me that the nachos were not actually gluten-free. The chips had cross contamination in the fryer. I couldn't believe it! It was even more frustrating because I had asked the right questions. Thankfully, something like this hasn't happened to me again.

What has been the biggest change since you became gluten free?

Every year, it becomes easier to follow a gluten-free diet! It's more straightforward to find gluten-free foods. Supermarkets and stores now have gluten-free sections, and food labeling has gotten better. Products market themselves to the gluten-free consumer. Some brands have even modified their ingredients in order to make their products gluten-free.

The restaurant scene has become more sensitive to people who follow a gluten-free diet. Some restaurants have menus that indicate which items are gluten-free, and this definitely wasn't the case seven years ago. Waiters are usually well-versed in how to accommodate dietary needs, unlike a few years ago when the majority of waiters didn't even know what gluten was.

In ten years, a gluten free diet will be...

Even more widespread. I see the gluten-free world continuing down the path of increased awareness. I've ate at nearly 70 completely gluten-free eateries, and I expect to see even more 100% gluten-free eateries in the future. I predict that the number of people who go gluten-free will keep on multiplying. After all, gluten-free food truly tastes good now, and it's a healthier way to live.

What is the best advice you received?

Make something people want.

What is the best way for people to connect with you?

Instagram: @glutenfree.followme Twitter: @glutenfreefm
Facebook: Gluten Free Follow Me glutenfreefollowme.com

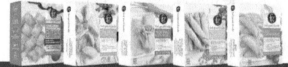
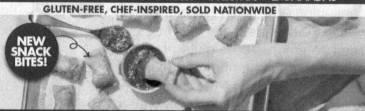

Best Gluten Free Frozen Pancake & Waffle Brands

10th Annual Gluten-Free Awards:

1st Place Winner: Van's Gluten Free Waffles

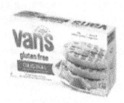

2nd Place Winner: Trader Joe's Gluten-Free Waffles

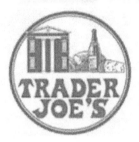

3rd Place Winner: Nature's Path Homestyle Frozen Waffle

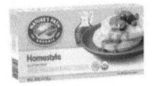

Other Great Products:

Kashi Gluten Free Waffles

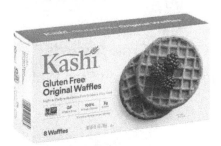

Know Foods Gluten Free Waffles

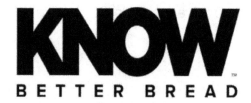

DID YOU KNOW?

GLUTEN CAN'T BE DIGESTED BY HUMAN BODY (LONG CHAIN AMINO ACID)

Quoted from:
17th International Celiac Disease
Symposium in New Delhi, India

Meet Michael Frolichstein

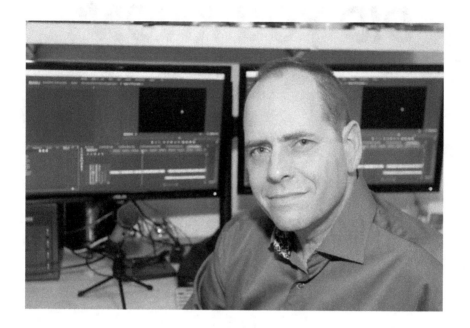

How long have you been gluten free?

10 years

Do you have any other dietary restrictions?

No

What has been your biggest challenge thus far?

By far the biggest challenge has to do with being social around food. I have to eat before going to parties and other get togethers.

Where is your favorite place to eat?

I have a few, but my favorite would be Wildfire. They have a number of locations in the Chicagoland area. It's a classic steakhouse style restaurant that has a substantial gluten free menu and excellent protocols in place to make sure the food is safe.

Do you have any gluten related pet peeves?

My biggest pet peeve is that so many people can't wrap their minds around cross contamination. I still get strange looks and eye rolls when avoiding gluten free foods in certain situations because of the risk of cross contact due to the circumstances.

Do you have any relatives are close friends that are gluten free?

Yes, there are 3 of us in my family with celiac (my daughter and nephew). My wife and her mother also went gluten free due to Hashimoto's disease and they feel much better.

Do you have a gluten horror story?

You bet I do. It coincidentally happened right around Halloween. We were making tacos and using a brand of tortillas that we thought at the time only made the corn variety. Midway through dinner my daughter commented on the taste and texture being different than what she was used to. My wife and my eyes met in horror, and I ran to the kitchen to confirm that they were indeed wheat tortillas. We are as diligent as one can be so my guilt over this was beyond belief. I had a terrible night and ended up passing out (after throwing up), but got through it. It was the only time, to my knowledge, in the past 10 years that I knowingly consumed a gluten containing product. It is a good reminder to always double and triple check items.

What has been the biggest change since you became gluten free?

It took me a while, but I feel better overall. The level of daily anxiety and stress that permeated my life took so much energy to contain. While living a gluten free life is not always easy or convenient, I feel so much better and less stressed by getting my health back. I find it amazing that I was able to function as well as I did before diagnosis, as I was experiencing symptoms from as early as age thirteen.

In ten years, a gluten free diet will be...

Better understood...or at least that is my hope! In the 10 years since I was diagnosed the awareness has been growing exponentially so I believe we as a society are on the right track. There may also be real treatments by then that, while maybe not allowing those with celiac to eat gluten, will hopefully allow us to not worry as much about cross contamination.

What is the best advice you received?

Stay the course. There are those people who feel better after a week of going gluten free, but the majority of us take much longer (due to the amount of damage). I was given this advice when I was diagnosed and I never strayed from the gluten free diet. When I meet people who are newly diagnosed with celiac disease and don't feel like they are getting better on the diet, I tell them to be patient.

What is the best way for people to connect with you?

They can email me at info@celiacproject.com or message me on Facebook, twitter or instagram @CeliacProject

Best Gluten Free Granola

10th Annual Gluten-Free Awards:

1st Place Winner: Kind Healthy Grains Clusters, Oats and Honey with Toasted Coconut Granola, Gluten Free

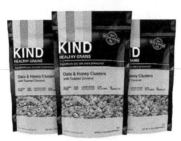

2nd Place Winner: Back to Nature Gluten-Free Vanilla Almond Agave Granola

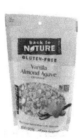

3rd Place Winner: Purely Elizabeth Ancient Grain Granola, Original

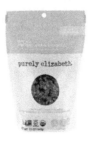

Other Great Products:

ALDI: liveGfree Gluten Free Granola - Apple Almond Honey

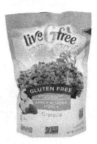

ALDI: liveGfree Gluten Free Granola - Raisin Almond Honey

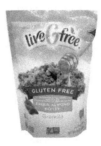

Purely Elizabeth Ancient Grain Granola, Original

Bubba's Fine Foods Bourbon Vanilla UnGranola

Goodness Grainless Granola Chocolate Cardamom

Autumn's Gold Grain Free Granola

Lidl Organic, Gluten Free Crunchy Granola

CELIAC SURVEY

We polled over 400 people with celiac disease with the intent to make you feel not so alone.

Do you have a dedicated gluten free toaster in your kitchen?

74% Yes

26% No

Presented by The 2020 Gluten Free Buyers Guide

YOU'RE NOT ALONE

Best Gluten Free Ice Cream Cones

10th Annual Gluten-Free Awards:

1st Place Winner: Joy Gluten-Free Sugar Ice Cream Cones

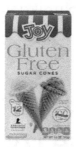

2nd Place Winner: Joy Gluten-Free Ice Cream Cones Cake Cups

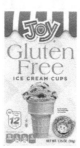

3rd Place Winner: Let's Do Organic Ice Cream Cones, Gluten Free

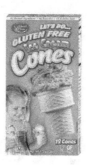

Other Great Products:

Goldbaum's Gluten Free Ice Cream Cone

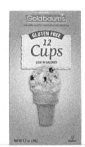

Edward & Sons Trading Co Cones, Sugar, Gluten Free

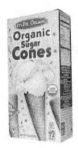

Barkat Gluten Free Waffle Ice Cream Cones

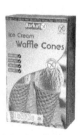

Meet Chrystal Carver

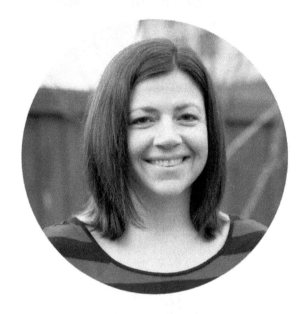

How long have you been gluten free?

10 years

Do you have any other dietary restrictions?

None

What has been your biggest challenge thus far?

Helping people understand that foods that are naturally gluten free can become contaminated during processing.

Where is your favorite place to eat?

I love a restaurant near me called Andina. For a quick bite to eat I like chipotle.

Do you have any gluten related pet peeves?

I can't stand it when people tell me that they are gluten free and only eat gluten a few times a week. Either you eat gluten free or you don't.

Do you have any relatives are close friends that are gluten free?

We recently found out that several of my relatives are Celiac. Also my husbands sister is Celiac. A few of my friends were also recently diagnosed.

Do you have a gluten horror story?

If I do, it was so bad that I blocked it from memory. I've accidentally taken bites, but nothing crazy.

What has been the biggest change since you became gluten free?

I no longer have brain fog. I feel more alive and more awake. Also, my digestive system is a lot happier.

In ten years, a gluten free diet will be...

even better tasting than it is today. We are continuing to develop recipes and products to have great textures and flavors. As we continue to learn we will adjust and create even better options.

What is the best advice you received?

Do what makes you feel the best inside and out.

What is the best way for people to connect with you?

You can find me at www.glutenfreepalate.com

Best Gluten Free Jerky

10th Annual Gluten-Free Awards:

1st Place Winner: OLD WISCONSIN Beef Snack Sticks

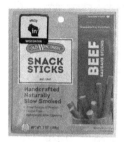

2nd Place Winner: Krave Sweet Chipotle Beef Jerky

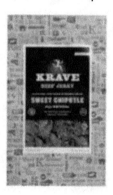

3rd Place Winner: EPIC Bison and Bacon Bites

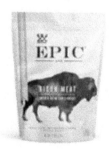

Other Great Products:

Perky Jerky 100% Grass-Fed Beef Teriyaki

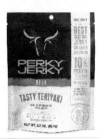

Oberto Spicy Sweet Beef Jerky

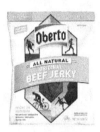

Nick's Sticks 100% Grass-Fed Beef Snack Sticks - Gluten Free

Country Archer Grass Fed Original Beef Jerky

The New Primal Sea Salt Beef Thins

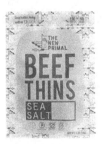

Katie's Carolina Reaper Spicy Beef Jerky-GLUTEN FREE

Best Gluten Free Macaroni and Cheese

10th Annual Gluten-Free Awards:

1st Place Winner: Amy's Gluten Free Frozen Mac & Cheese

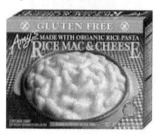

2nd Place Winner: ALDI: liveGfree Gluten Free Shells & Cheese

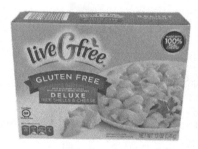

3rd Place Winner: Annie's Organic Vegan Macaroni and Cheese, Elbows & Creamy Sauce, Gluten Free Pasta

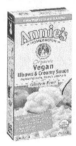

Other Great Products:

Trader Joe's Gluten Free Mac & Cheese

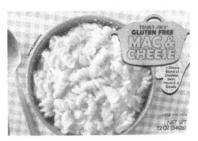

Pamela's Products Gourmet Gluten Free High Protein Pasta Meal with Real Cheese, Mac N' Cheese

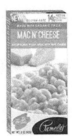

Banza Chickpea Pasta – High Protein Gluten Free Mac & Cheese

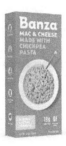

CELIAC SURVEY

We polled over 400 people with celiac disease
with the intent to make you feel not so alone.

Do you
try to keep your diagnosis
a secret or do you share
your story?

50% Share
49% It depends
1% Keep it secret

Presented by The 2020 Gluten Free Buyers Guide

YOU'RE NOT ALONE

Meet Jenna Drew Dancy

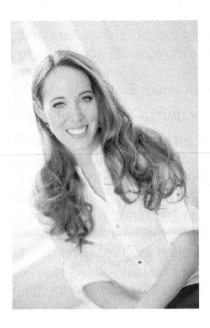

How long have you been gluten free?

10 years

Do you have any other dietary restrictions?

My stomach is unruly - and I find that my body performs at it's best when I fuel it with real foods, smoothies, and cold-pressed juices. Eggplant is a total no-go for me!

What has been your biggest challenge thus far?

There was a steep learning curve as I started to learn more about gluten free living. I went from eating anything and everything to having to closely decode ingredient labels because there wasn't any labeling laws to declare the Top 8 Allergens. My new challenge with two young children is learning how to manage their relationship with food until knowing whether or not they have Celiac Disease. We have a gluten free home to create a safe haven and avoid cross contamination.

Where is your favorite place to eat?

I do a lot of cooking when I am at home. I've traveled over 75,000 miles the last few years, and it is fun to find new restaurants around the world that are dedicated gluten free restaurants or knowledgeable about Celiac Disease. After living in NYC for almost 10 years, I love any excuse I can get to eat at Senza Gluten or Bistango in NYC.

Do you have any gluten related pet peeves?

It is frustrating when you see people who don't necessarily have to be gluten free (it's more of a choice for them) order gluten free at a restaurant and then when someone else at the table has gluten-filled food, they will ask for a bite. No wonder why untrained staff at restaurants don't always take a precaution when someone orders gluten free without sharing that it is from a medical condition. I used to HATE telling waitstaff that I had Celiac Disease, but now I feel it's important to share, so they can see the difference between a want and a need to be gluten free.

Do you have any relatives are close friends that are gluten free?

Yes, my mom is gluten free because she has Celiac Disease.

Do you have a gluten horror story?

Most of my horror stories have actually been from dining experiences at the homes of family and friends. I remember eating a friend's house that needed to gluten free as well so I felt comfortable. However, not everything at her house was gluten free. When she served dinner she mistakenly gave us both the flour taco shells full of gluten! After just a bite, I knew that it didn't taste gluten free.

What has been the biggest change since you became gluten free?

It took me 5 years on a gluten free diet to feel better. I dealt with an unruly stomach, constant fatigue, brain fog, focus issues, migraines, and heighten stress levels. It wasn't until I ditched most of the processed gluten free foods that my gut

Other Great Products:

yum.

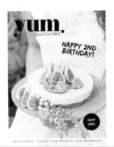

Delight Gluten Free

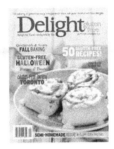

GFF Magazine

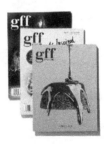

Allergic Living Magazine

Best Gluten Free Mobile Apps

10th Annual Gluten-Free Awards:

1st Place Winner: Find Me Gluten Free

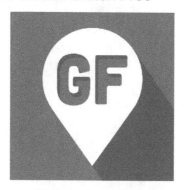

2nd Place Winner: The Gluten Free Scanner

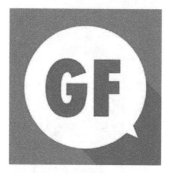

3rd Place Winner: GF Plate

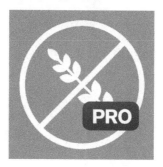

Other Great Apps:

Grain or No Grain

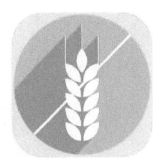

Now Find Gluten Free

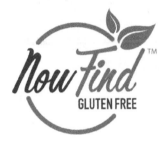

Dedicated Gluten Free

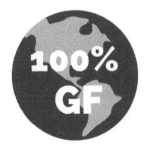

Grain or No Grain

Meet Michelle Palin

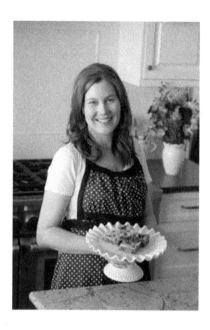

How long have you been gluten free?

9 years

Do you have any other dietary restrictions?

I have a number of foods I need to avoid due to IBS and gastroparesis.

What has been your biggest challenge thus far?

No one invites me/our family over anymore. I wish they would and just let me bring my own food for myself (or eat before I come).

Where is your favorite place to eat?

New Cascadia in Portland, OR.

Do you have any gluten related pet peeves?

When people say to me, "I eat gluten-free sometimes, just because it's healthier."

Do you have any relatives are close friends that are gluten free?

Many gluten-free friends! I've met so many other people with celiac that have become great friends.

Do you have a gluten horror story?

not really one to share.

What has been the biggest change since you became gluten free?

Well probably my weight! I went from 20 lbs. underweight pre-diagnosis to 25 lbs. overweight now.

In ten years, a gluten free diet will be...

Probably quite similar. But my hope is that there will be a cure for celiac by then so not as many of us will have to avoid gluten 100 percent.

What is the best advice you received?

Don't be afraid to get in the kitchen and learn to bake gluten-free. You really don't have to miss out on your favorite foods - you can make them all. (well, except croissants!)

What is the best way for people to connect with you?

Everyone can find my recipes and tips on my blog: https://mygluten-freekitchen.com/ I love to interact with my readers on Facebook the most, more than other social media. My Facebook is: https://www.facebook.com/MyGlutenfreeKitchenblog/

Best Gluten Free Muffin Mix

10th Annual Gluten-Free Awards:

1st Place Winner: Krusteaz Gluten Free Blueberry Muffin Mix

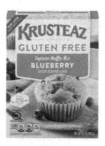

2nd Place Winner: King Arthur Gluten Free Muffin Mix

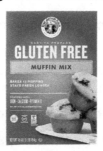

3rd Place Winner: gfJules Muffin Mix

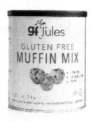

Other Great Products:

Simple Mills Naturally Gluten-Free Almond Flour Mix, Pumpkin Muffin & Bread

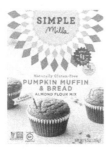

Namaste Foods Gluten Free Muffin Mix

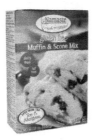

Cooggies Gluten Free Baking Mix, Bare Muffin

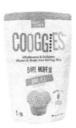

Vitacost Blueberry Muffin Mix - Non-GMO and Gluten Free

Good Dee's Lemon Muffin Mix - Gluten Free

CELIAC SURVEY

We polled over 400 people with celiac disease
with the intent to make you feel not so alone.

Does your family support your gluten free lifestyle?

97% Yes

3% No

Presented by The 2020 Gluten Free Buyers Guide

YOU'RE NOT ALONE

Best Gluten Free Munchies

10th Annual Gluten-Free Awards:

1st Place Winner: Angie's BOOMCHICKAPOP Sweet & Salty Kettle Corn Popcorn

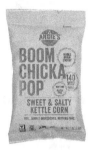

2nd Place Winner: Gratify Gluten Free Everything Thins Pretzels

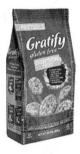

3rd Place Winner: Three Bakers' Honey Graham Snackers

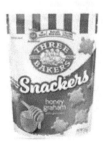

Other Great Products:

Three Bakers Chocolate Chip Snackers

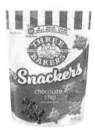

Three Bakers Chocolate Chocolate Chip Snackers

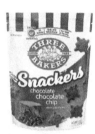

Evolved Chocolate - Organic Almond Butter Cups

Safely Delicious®🛇 Minty Bites®🛇

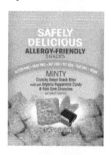

Quinn Snacks Non-GMO and Gluten Free Pretzels, Classic Sea Salt

The Real Coconut, Himalayan Pink Salt, Gluten Free Coconut Flour Tortilla Chips

Sunfood Superfoods Macadamia Nuts

Meet Jules Shepard

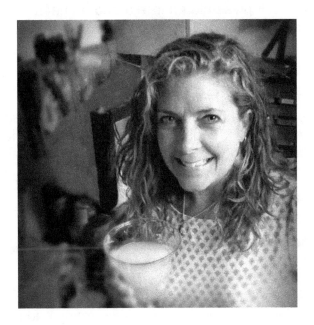

How long have you been gluten free?

20 years!

Do you have any other dietary restrictions?

lactose intolerant & vegetarian/pescatarian

What has been your biggest challenge thus far?

Eating out is still a challenge, as more and more restaurants offer "gluten free menus" but don't understand how to truly serve safe gluten free food from a co-mingled kitchen.

Where is your favorite place to eat?

Any Thai or Indian restaurant! LOL Ok, I'm a little pickier than that, and I always do my homework to be sure I can order safely, but generally Thai and Indian restaurants tend to be easier to order safe gluten free food than most.

Do you have any gluten related pet peeves?

It is super frustrating that so many manufacturers and restaurants offer "gluten free" food that is so mediocre, or just plain bad. It gives gluten free a bad name! It doesn't have to be that way - gluten free food can and should be amazing. Stop compromising, people!

Do you have any relatives are close friends that are gluten free?

My mother and grandfather both have celiac disease as well. I also have several friends whose children have celiac disease and one good friend who lives close and has celiac. I love "gifting" my recipe tests to them after photo shoots.

Do you have a gluten horror story?

Once a restaurant served me something with soy sauce and after I tasted a couple bites I asked again if they were sure there was no soy sauce. They double checked and then apologized that the chef had mistakenly put soy sauce in it. I was sick for 3 weeks - I was so miserable. I won't order that dish again, no matter where I am -- too many bad memories.

What has been the biggest change since you became gluten free?

The amount of gluten free food available in stores and restaurants (whether safe or good or not); when I went gluten free, no one even knew what gluten was! My, how times have changed!

In ten years, a gluten free diet will be...

Mainstream!

What is the best advice you received?

To share my learnings with others. I truly felt like I was inventing the "how to live gluten free" wheel, and I was encouraged to not keep it to myself! I wrote one book, and then another, and then another, started a blog, hosted a podcast, recorded hundreds of gluten free videos and have traveled all over the country teaching and speaking about baking and living gluten free. It has been so rewarding for me to share and to help others.

What is the best way for people to connect with you?

Through my blog - gfJules.com or social media @gfJules (Facebook, Pinterest, Instagram) @THEgfJules (Twitter)

Best Gluten Free National Restaurant Chains

10th Annual Gluten-Free Awards:

1st Place Winner: Chick-fil-A

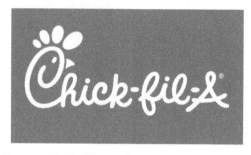

2nd Place Winner: P.F. Chang's

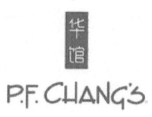

3rd Place Winner: Chipotle

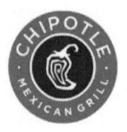

Other Great Products:

Red Robin

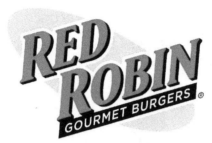

Outback Steakhouse

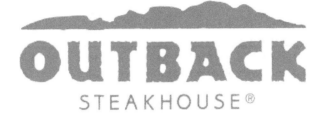

Jersey Mike's

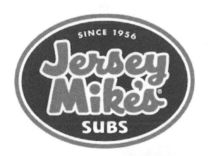

California Pizza Kitchen

The Bonefish Grill

True Food Kitchen

Best Gluten Free New Products

10th Annual Gluten-Free Awards:

1st Place Winner: Canyon Bakehouse Honey Whole Grain English Muffins

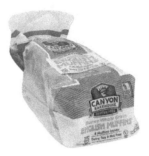

2nd Place Winner Goodie Girl Cookies Cinnamon Brown Sugar Gluten Free Breakfast Biscuits

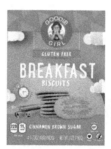

3rd Place Winner: MadeGood Chocolate Chip Soft Baked Cookies

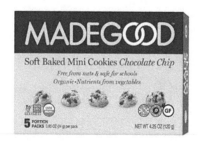

Other Great Products:

Safely Delicious®️ Lemony Bites®️

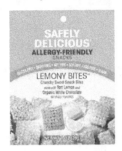

Three Bakers Large Slice Whole Grain White

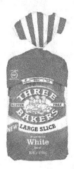

Emmys, Cookies Organic Dark Cacao Coconut

Three Bakers Large Slice Golden Flax

Autumn's Gold Maple Grain Free Granola

Tasterie - Allergen Friendly "Grab 'N Go" Care Pack

Palacios Alimentaction - Organic Spanish Chorizo

Palacios Alimentaction - Mild Spanish Chorizo

CELIAC SURVEY

We polled over 400 people with celiac disease
with the intent to make you feel not so alone.

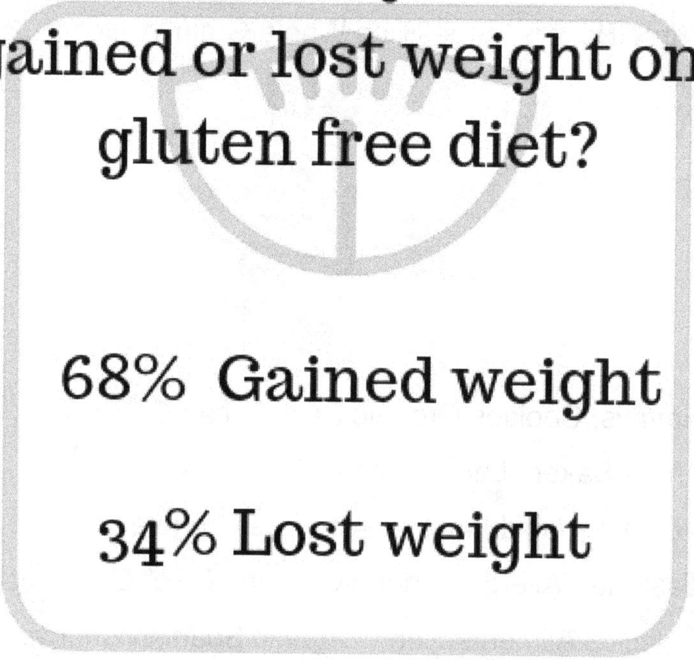

Have you gained or lost weight on a gluten free diet?

68% Gained weight

34% Lost weight

Presented by The 2020 Gluten Free Buyers Guide

YOU'RE NOT ALONE

Meet Lori Miller

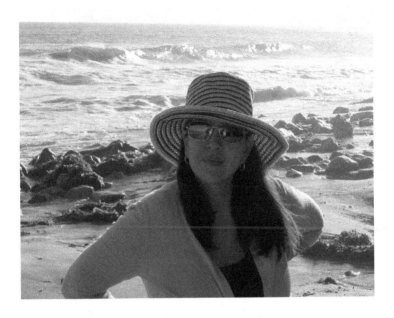

How long have you been gluten free?

Since November 1999, so almost 10 years

Do you have any other dietary restrictions?

I have a dairy allergy.

What has been your biggest challenge thus far?

Eating out is very difficult because most gluten-free options still have dairy.

Where is your favorite place to eat?

At home.

Do you have any gluten related pet peeves?

The constant 'victimology' mythology that living with Celiac Disease makes us all victims. I see too many posts on social media with whiny comments about feeling victimized. I will never consider myself a victim. I consider my diagnosis a blessing because I now know what I need to do for my body to feel good!

Do you have any relatives are close friends that are gluten free?

A few.

Do you have a gluten horror story?

None as of yet, and hopefully never!

What has been the biggest change since you became gluten free?

Eating out is a struggle, so when my husband and I travel, we need to rent places with kitchen so we can prepare our food.

In ten years, a gluten free diet will be...

Mainstream and common.

What is the best advice you received?

To nourish my body with healthy gluten-free options!

What is the best way for people to connect with you?

Via email: glutenfreeglobalicious@gmail.com

Best Gluten Free Non-Profits

10th Annual Gluten-Free Awards:

1st Place Winner: Celiac Disease Foundation (CDF)

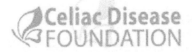

2nd Place Winner: Gluten Intolerance Group of North America (GIG)

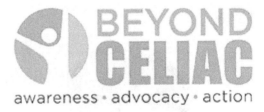

3rd Place Winner: Beyond Celiac

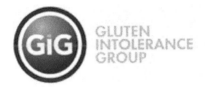

Other Great Non-Profits:

Celiac Support Association (CSA) (formerly Celiac Sprue Association)

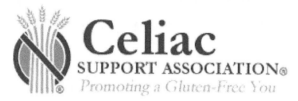

National Celiac Disease Society (NCDS)

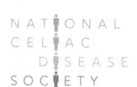

The Rachel Way

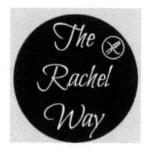

Cutting Costs for Celiacs Food Equality Initiative

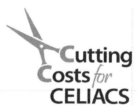

DID YOU KNOW?

1:2 IN THE UNITED STATES WILL TRY A GLUTEN-FREE DIET THIS YEAR

Quoted from:
17th International Celiac Disease
Symposium in New Delhi, India

Best Gluten Free Online Resources

10th Annual Gluten-Free Awards:

1st Place Winner: GfJules.com

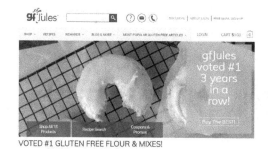

VOTED #1 GLUTEN FREE FLOUR & MIXES!

2nd Place Winner: Celiac.org

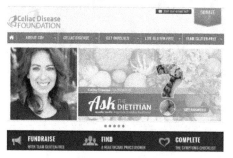

3rd Place Winner: GlutenFreeWatchDog.org

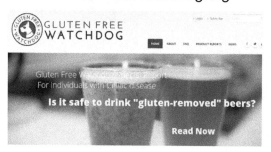

Other Great Websites:

Beyondceliac.org

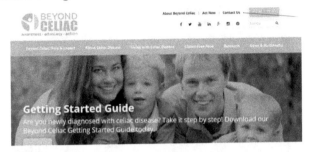

Glutenfreefollowme.com

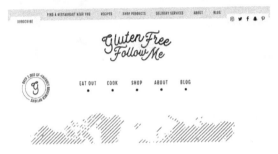

Gluten.org

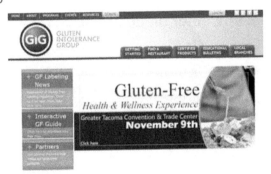

CeliacCentral.org

GlutenfreeGlobalicious.com

certifiedglutenpractitioner.com

researchgate.net

buenqamino.com

Meet Taylor Miller

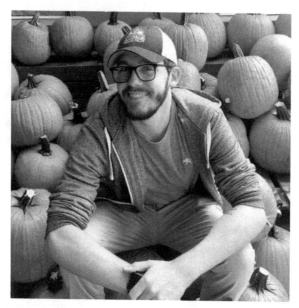

How long have you been gluten free?

8 years

Do you have any other dietary restrictions?

Pescatarian

What has been your biggest challenge thus far?

Dining out gluten-free has always been a challenge but it has gotten easier as more restaurants add options.

Where is your favorite place to eat?

BareBurger

Do you have any gluten related pet peeves?

People who say "can't you have just a little".

Do you have any relatives are close friends that are gluten free?

Yes, my mother and many blogger friends!

Do you have a gluten horror story?

Unfortunately, there's been a few times where I ordered something gluten-free at a restaurant and after I get half way through the meal, the waiter comes out and says they made a mistake and gave me the gluten full meal.

Q9What has been the biggest change since you became gluten free?

I have become much more aware of my body and what I put in it. Socializing became harder but got easier over time. I just had to take control of my own diet and health.

In ten years, a gluten free diet will be...

Even more well-known and advocated for among those with celiac disease.

What is the best advice you received?

Don't beat yourself up if you make mistakes when gluten-free. Everyone does and just like anything else, mistakes are a part of life.

What is the best way for people to connect with you?

Social media! Any platform including twitter, Instagram, and Facebook @halelifetaylor

Best Gluten Free Online Stores

10th Annual Gluten-Free Awards:

1st Place Winner: Amazon

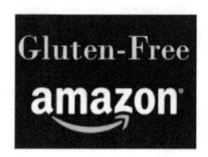

2nd Place Winner: Thrive Market

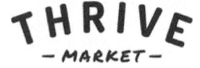

3rd Place Winner: Gluten Free Mall

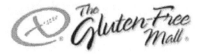

Other Great Stores:

Vitacost

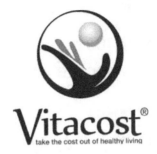

Walmart Online

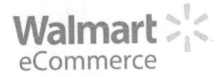

Target Online

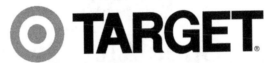

Nuts.com

Jet.com

CELIAC SURVEY

We polled over 400 people with celiac disease with the intent to make you feel not so alone.

What food do you miss the most?

#1 Pizza

#2 Specialty Breads

#3 Various Pastries

Presented by The 2020 Gluten Free Buyers Guide

YOU'RE NOT ALONE

Best Gluten Free Pancake and Waffle Mixes

10th Annual Gluten-Free Awards:

1st Place Winner: Bisquick Gluten Free

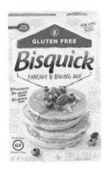

2nd Place Winner: Pamela's Products Gluten Free Baking and Pancake Mix

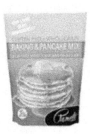

3rd Place Winner: gfJules Pancake & Waffle Mix

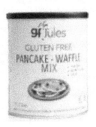

Other Great Products:

Kodiak Cakes Gluten Free Protein Pancake Flapjack & Waffle Baking Mix

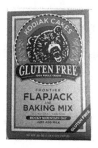

Birch Benders Gluten Free Pancake & Waffle Mix

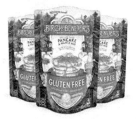

Enjoy Life Foods, Gluten Free Pancake And Waffle Mix With Ancient Grains

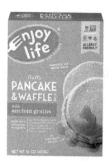

Better Batter Gluten Free Pancake and Biscuit Mix

Whole Note Gluten Free Baking Mix, Buttermilk Pancake Mix

Meet Maureen Stanley

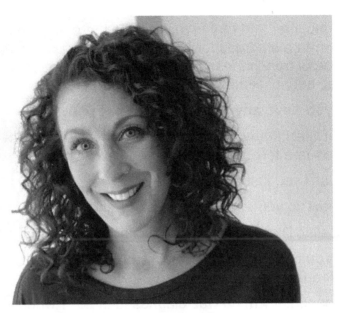

How long have you been gluten free?

I was diagnosed in 2005 after several misdiagnoses including Ulcerative Colitis and "pregnancy-related".

Do you have any other dietary restrictions?

Quinoa and cranberries are off-limits. The effects are similar to being glutened, but not as extreme. I'm also a vegetarian by choice (since 1991).

What has been your biggest challenge thus far?

Losing some of my spontaneity and having a bit of what I like to call "food anxiety". So much of our lives are connected to food. Social gatherings, holidays, and travel all need planning. The last thing I want to do is spend Thanksgiving in the bathroom.

Where is your favorite place to eat?

Anywhere that is a 100% dedicated gluten-free restaurant or bakery makes my heart and belly happy!

Fox and Sons Fancy Corn Dogs at Reading Terminal in Philadelphia is beyond amazing. Every single food they serve is gluten-free.

My daughter and I try to make a trip there every month for a gluten-free smorgasbord of funnel cake, fried cheese curds, hand-cut french fries, and fried faux-reos. Not the healthiest meal, but absolutely delicious.

Do you have any gluten related pet peeves?

Most likely many of the same pet peeves the rest of us gluten-free folk have. When people exclaim:

1) Can't you just take it off the roll?

2) How do you live without cookies and donuts?

3) Celiac Disease isn't real (this one really gets me going)

Do you have any relatives are close friends that are gluten free?

My daughter Emma was diagnosed in 2011 when she was in fourth grade. While I'll always feel guilty for passing my bad genetics on to her, I feel extremely lucky to have someone so close to me that "gets it". Our mother/daughter time together often includes enjoying a gluten-free meal together.

Do you have a gluten horror story?

September 2015 will go down in infamy in my gluten-free life. To set the stage, I have a one-hour window if I'm glutened.

Our local pizza place began offering gluten-free pizza. It was not a dedicated facility, but they claimed to be knowledgeable of Celiac Disease.

Excitedly, I ordered a gluten-free pizza for takeout. At home, I gobbled several pieces of pizza down. Then I decided to head out clothes shopping. It's a half-hour drive to the store and I'm looking forward to some serious retail therapy.

About ten minutes into shopping, I start feeling extremely nauseous. My stomach begins rumbling. I'm sweating like I've just run a marathon.

That's when I realize I've been glutened.

I know what's coming, so I exit the store as quickly as possible. I make it as far as the parking lot when I begin to projectile vomit. Literally Exorcist style. Once the puking starts, it doesn't stop for hours. I can only imagine the parking lot video surveillance.

It turns out the pizza place gave us a regular gluten-filled pizza. Now, I'm sure you're wondering "how the heck does Maureen not know the difference between a gluten-free and gluten-filled pizza?"

In my defense, the pizza had all of the delightful qualities of a gluten-free pizza: small in size and fairly unappetizing in taste.

The terrible part was that I was so ill I ended up in the Emergency Room and spent several days bedridden.

The positive part was that I did not poop my pants. I was also reminded of an important life lesson as a Celiac. Go with your gut - if the food doesn't look gluten-free, then ask. If the business doesn't provide a clear explanation of their gluten-free food prep process, then don't eat there.

It's just not worth it.

What has been the biggest change since you became gluten free?

My eyeglass prescription due to reading extremely tiny labels. In all seriousness, I'm SO much more aware of what we're putting into and onto our bodies.

In ten years, a gluten free diet will be...

Tastier. When I was diagnosed in 2005, the cardboard box the gluten-free food came in tasted better than the food inside. With each passing year, the gluten-free food industry has grown in both options and taste. I can't wait to find out what gluten-free bread will taste like in 2029!

What is the best advice you received?

To speak up and be your own advocate. Yes, it can be hard at times (especially if you don't like to draw attention to yourself or rock the boat), but it's an opportunity to educate others. It doesn't make you high-maintenance, it shows that you care about yourself, your health, and well-being. Because you certainly deserve it!

What is the best way for people to connect with you?

I love hearing from others in the gluten-free community and feel privileged in all that they share with me. Yes, even those "special" stories about how they were terribly glutened and what happened afterward. You can get in touch with me via:

E-mail Maureen@holdthegluten.com Website holdthegluten.com Facebook, Instagram and Twitter @holdthegluten

Best Gluten Free Pastas

10th Annual Gluten-Free Awards:

1st Place Winner: Barilla Gluten Free Rotini

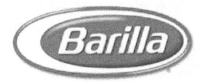

2nd Place Winner: ALDI: liveGfree

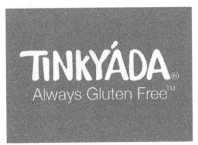

3rd Place Winner: Tinkyada

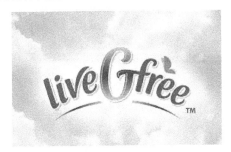

Other Great Products:

Ronzoni

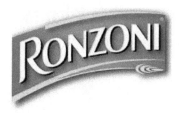

Jovial

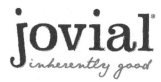

Ancient Harvest

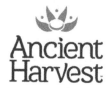

Cappello's

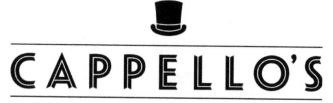

Le Veneziane

Bionaturae

Rummo

Best Gluten Free Pie Crust

10th Annual Gluten-Free Awards:

1st Place Winner: King Arthur Flour Gluten Free Pie Crust Mix

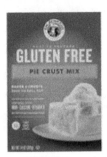

2nd Place Winner: Trader Joe's Frozen Gluten Free Pie Crust

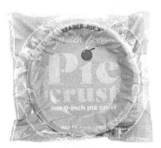

3rd Place Winner: Midel Graham Cracker Crust

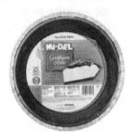

Other Great Products:

Wholly Wholesome Gluten Free 9" Pie Shells

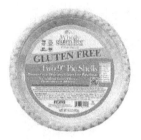

Cup4Cup Gluten-Free Pie Crust Mix

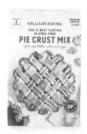

Williams Sonoma Gluten-Free Pie Crust Mix

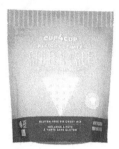

Inspiration Mix Gluten Free Pie Crust Mix

CELIAC SURVEY

We polled over 400 people with celiac disease
with the intent to make you feel not so alone.

Do you think the celebrity
/ Hollywood gluten free
trend helped or hurt those
with Celiac Disease?

57% Hurt

43% Helped

Presented by The 2020 Gluten Free Buyers Guide

YOU'RE NOT ALONE

Best Gluten Free Pizza Crust

10th Annual Gluten-Free Awards:

1st Place Winner: Bob's Red Mill Pizza Crust Mix

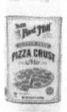

2nd Place Winner: gfJules Pizza Crust Mix

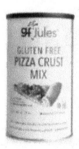

3rd Place Winner: Pamela's Products Gluten Free Pizza Crust Mix

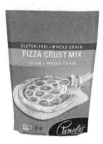

Other Great Products:

Betty Crocker Gluten Free Pizza Crust Mix

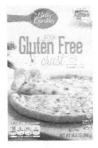

Chebe - Gluten Free Pizza Crust Mix

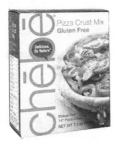

Simple Mills Pizza Dough Mix

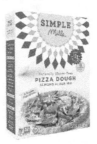

Stonewall Kitchen Gluten-free Herbed Pizza Crust Mix

Gluten Free Prairie Our Best Pizza & Flatbread Mix

Cooqi Gluten Free Pizza & Pita Mix

Best Gluten Free Podcasts

10th Annual Gluten-Free Awards:

1st Place Winner: Gluten Free You & Me

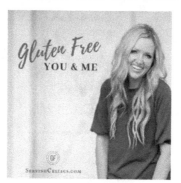

2nd Place Winner: The Celiac Project Podcast

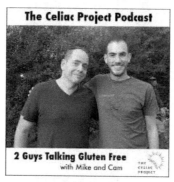

3rd Place Winner: The Gluten Free Baking Show

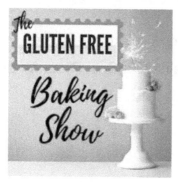

Other Great Gluten Free Podcasts

Travel Gluten Free

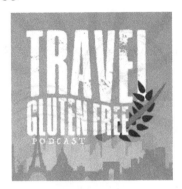

The Gluten Free Guide

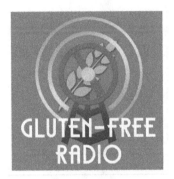

Gluten Free RN

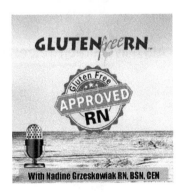

Best Gluten Free Pretzels

10th Annual Gluten-Free Awards:

1st Place Winner: Snyder's of Hanover Gluten Free Pretzel Sticks

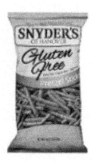

2nd Place Winner: Glutino Pretzel Twists, Salted

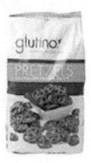

3rd Place Winner: ALDI liveGfree Pretzel Sticks

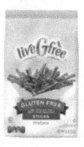

Other Great Products:

Utz Gluten Free Pretzel Sticks

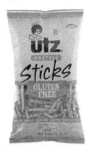

Quinn, Peanut Butter & Chocolate Filled Pretzels

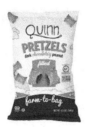

Gratify Gluten Free Pretzel Thins Sesame Seed

Snack Factory Gluten Free Minis Pretzel Crisps

Tonya's Gluten Free Soft Pretzels

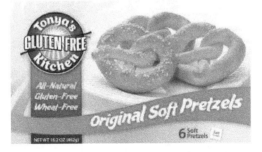

Good Health Inc. Gluten Free Sea Salt Pretzels

FitJoy Grain Free Pretzels, Gluten Free

CELIAC SURVEY

We polled over 400 people with celiac disease with the intent to make you feel not so alone.

Have people made fun of the gluten free diet in front of you?

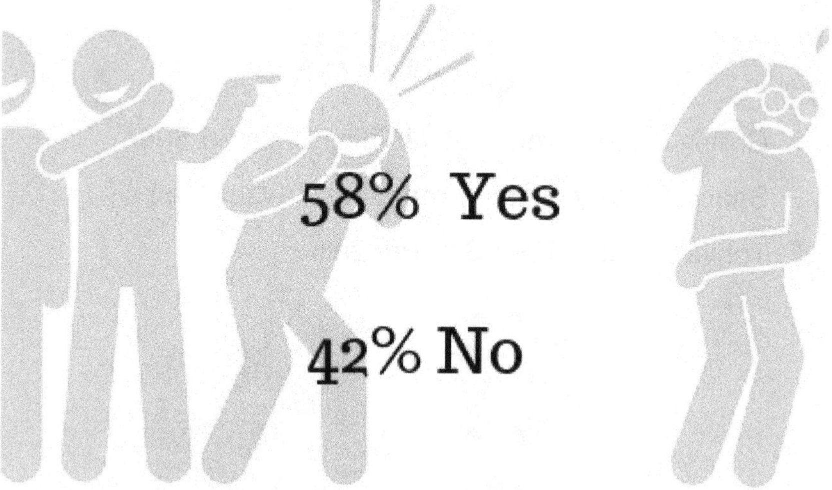

58% Yes

42% No

Presented by The 2020 Gluten Free Buyers Guide

YOU'RE NOT ALONE

Best Gluten Free Ready-Made Desserts

10th Annual Gluten-Free Awards:

1st Place Winner: Katz Gluten Free Chocolate Crème Filled Cupcakes

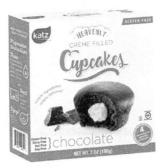

2nd Place Winner: Daiya New York Cheezecake

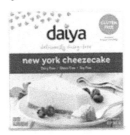

3rd Place Winner: Katz Gluten Free Vanilla Crème Cakes

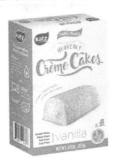

Other Great Products:

Hail Merry Chocolate Almond Butter Tart

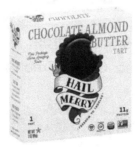

Chilly Cow - Brown Butter Salted Caramel

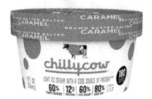

The Piping Gourmets Chocolate Mint Gluten-Free Whoopie Pies

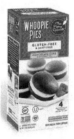

Safely Delicious®⎕ Dark Bites®⎕

Best Gluten Free Rolls

10th Annual Gluten-Free Awards:

1st Place Winner: Schär: Ciabatta Rolls

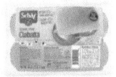

2nd Place Winner: Udi's Gluten Free Classic French Dinner Rolls

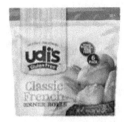

3rd Place Winner: Schär: Sub Sandwich Rolls

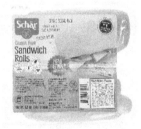

Other Great Products:

Three Bakers' Whole Grain Hoagie Roll

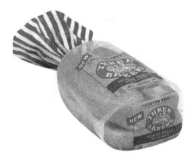

Bread SRSLY Gluten-Free Sourdough Sandwich Rolls

Katz Gluten Free Oat Rolls

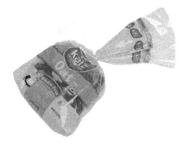

Bfree Gluten Free Rolls, Seeded Brown

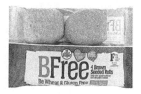

New Cascadia Traditionals Hoagie Rolls

Best Gluten Free Sauces

10th Annual Gluten-Free Awards:

1st Place Winner: San-J Organic Gluten Free Tamari Soy Sauce (Gold Label)

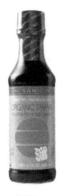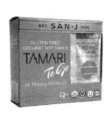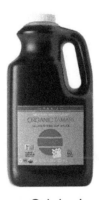

2nd Place Winner: Stubb's BBQ Sauce - Original

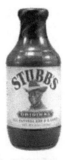

3rd Place Winner: Rao's Homemade Marinara Sauce

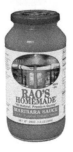

Other Great Products:

Francesco Rinaldi Three Cheese Hearty Pasta Sauce

Organic BBQ Sauce Original

Asian Fusion Gluten Free General Tso Sauce

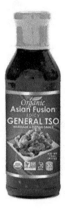

Dinosaur BBQ Honey Roasted Garlic Sauce

Saffron Road Lemongrass Basil Simmer Sauce

Claude's: Barbeque Brisket Marinade Sauce

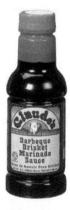

Blue Top Brand Cilantro Serrano Creamy Hot Sauce

CELIAC SURVEY

We polled over 400 people with celiac disease
with the intent to make you feel not so alone.

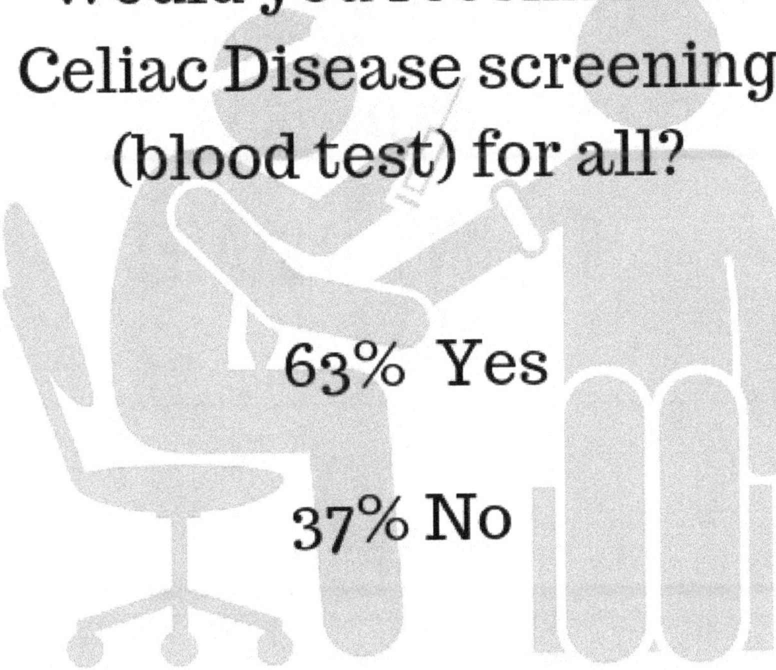

Would you recommend Celiac Disease screening (blood test) for all?

63% Yes

37% No

Presented by The 2020 Gluten Free Buyers Guide

YOU'RE NOT ALONE

DID YOU KNOW?

CELIAC DISEASE CASES DOUBLE EVERY 15 YEARS IN THE UNITED STATES

Quoted from:
17th International Celiac Disease
Symposium in New Delhi, India

Best Gluten Free Snack Bars

10th Annual Gluten-Free Awards:

1st Place Winner: KIND Bars, Caramel Almond and Sea Salt

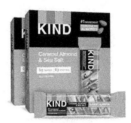

2nd Place Winner: Larabar - Peanut Butter Chocolate Chip

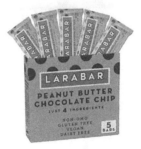

3rd Place Winner: Nature's Bakery Gluten Free Fig Bar, Blueberry Flavor

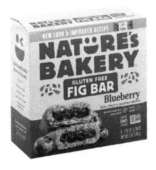

Other Great Products:

Enjoy Life Snack Bar - Coco Loco

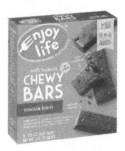

ALDI: liveGfree Gluten Free Chewy Bar: Very Berry

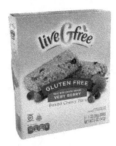

ALDI: liveGfree Gluten Free Chewy Bar: Caramel Apple

Nature's Bakery Gluten Free Fig Bar, Pomegranate Flavor

ONE Protein Bars, Birthday Cake

Caveman Foods Paleo-Friendly Nutrition Bar Dark
Chocolate Almond Coconut

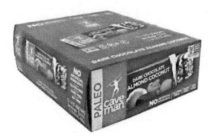

LivBar - Blueberry Vanilla Kale

Best Gluten Free Social Media Platforms

10th Annual Gluten-Free Awards:

1st Place Winner: Facebook

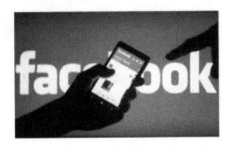

2nd Place Winner: Pinterest

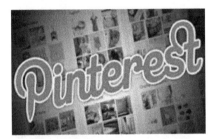

3rd Place Winner: Instagram

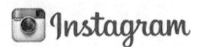

Other Great Social Media Platforms:

Twitter

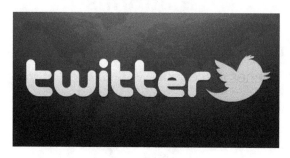

Freedible

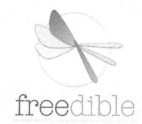

Meet-Up

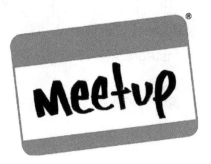

Linked In

Best Gluten Free Soups

10th Annual Gluten-Free Awards:

1st Place Winner: Progresso Soup Rich & Hearty New England Clam Chowder Soup Gluten Free

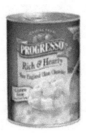

2nd Place Winner: Amy's Organic Thai Coconut Soup (Tom Kha Phak)

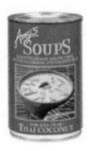

3rd Place Winner: Wolfgang Puck Organic Free Range Chicken with White & Wild Rice Soup

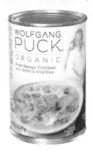

Other Great Products:

Gluten Free Cafe Chicken Noodle Soup

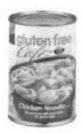

Boulder Organic Gluten Free Chicken Noodle Soup

Streit's Gluten Free Matzoh Ball Mix and Soup Mix

San-J White Miso Soup Envelopes

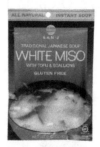

Dr McDougall's Gluten Free Rice Noodle Asian Soup, Sesame Chicken

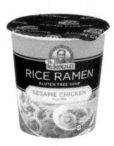

CELIAC SURVEY

We polled over 400 people with celiac disease
with the intent to make you feel not so alone.

Is it harder to date others
when you are on a gluten
free diet?

55% Yes

45% No

Presented by The 2020 Gluten Free Buyers Guide

YOU'RE NOT ALONE

Best Gluten Free Stuffing

10th Annual Gluten-Free Awards:

1st Place Winner: ALDI: liveGfree Gluten Free Chicken Stuffing

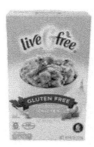

2nd Place Winner: Three Bakers' Herb Seasoned Stuffing Mix

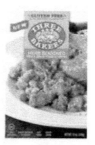

3rd Place Winner: Aleia's Gluten Free Savory Stuffing

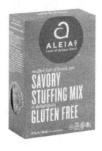

Other Great Products:

Ian's Natural Foods Gluten Free Savory Stuffing

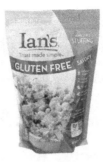

Williams Sonoma Gluten-Free Stuffing

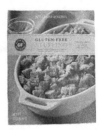

Gordon Rhodes - Gluten Free Sage and Onion Stuffing Mix

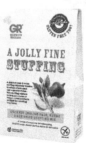

Best Gluten Free Summer Camps

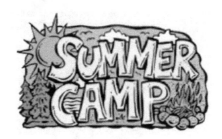

10th Annual Gluten-Free Awards:

1st Place Winner: The Great Gluten Escape at GilmontGilmer, Texas

2nd Place Winner: Camp Blue Spruce - Portland, OR

3rd Place Winner: Gluten-Free Overnight Camp Middleville, Michigan

Other Great Camps:

Gluten-Free Fun Camp Maple Lake, Minnesota

GIG (Gluten Intolerance Group) Kids Camp East Camp Kanata Wake Forest, North Carolina

Camp Celiac Strong - Hunt, NY

Camp Celiac Livermore, California

International Sports Training Camp Pocono Mountains, Pennsylvania

Camp Celiac North Scituate, Rhode Island

Camp Weekaneatit Warm Springs, Georgia

Gluten Detectives Camp (Day Camp)Bloomington, Minnesota

Appel Farm Arts Camp Elmer, New Jersey

CDF Camp Gluten-Free™ Camp Fire Camp Nawakwa San Bernardino Mountains, CA

Camp TAG - Williamstown, New Jersey

Timber Lake Camp Shandaken, New York

Camp Emerson Hinsdale, Massachusetts

Camp TAG Lebanon, Ohio at YMCA's Camp Kern.

GIG Kids Camp West Camp Sealth Vashon Island, Washington

Emma Kaufmann Camp Morgantown, West Virginia

Foundation for Children & Youth with Diabetes Camp UTADA West Jordan, Utah

Clear Creek Camp Green's Canyon, Utah (Serves Alpine School District children)

Camp Eagle Hill Elizaville, New York

Camp Silly-Yak Brigadoon Village Aylesford, Nova Scotia

Best Gluten Free Supplements

10th Annual Gluten-Free Awards:

1st Place Winner: Nature's Bounty Daily Multi

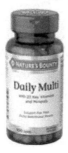

2nd Place Winner: Garden of Life Gluten Free Support

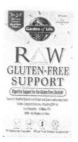

3rd Place Winner: Vega

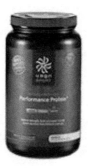

Other Great Products:

Olly

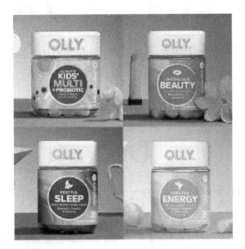

Enzymedica - Digest Gold with ATPro, Daily Digestive Support Supplement

MegaFood – Daily

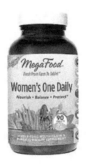

Jarrow - Organic Plant Protein Salted Caramel

Standard Process Whole Food Fiber

Silver Fern Ultimate Probiotic

Growing Naturals Rice Protein

E3 Advanced PlusProtein

CELIAC SURVEY

We polled over 400 people with celiac disease
with the intent to make you feel not so alone.

Do you attend any celiac support group meetings?

11% Yes

89% No

Presented by The 2020 Gluten Free Buyers Guide

YOU'RE NOT ALONE

Best Gluten Free Tortilla or Wrap

10th Annual Gluten-Free Awards:

1st Place Winner: La Tortilla Factory Gluten Free Ivory Teff Wraps

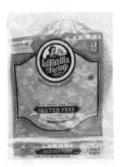

2nd Place Winner: Siete Almond Flour Grain Free Tortillas

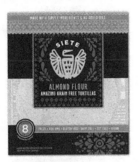

3rd Place Winner: Mikey's Tortillas

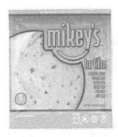

Other Great Products:

CAULIPOWER Original Cauliflower Tortilla

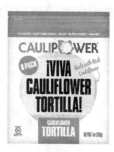

CAULIPOWER Grain Free Cauliflower Tortilla

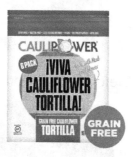

La Banderita Mini Taquito Corn Tortillas

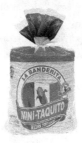

Julian Bakery Paleo Wraps

Mikey's Burritos

Raw Organic Spirulina Mini Veggie Wraps

NUCO Certified ORGANIC Paleo Gluten Free Vegan
Turmeric Coconut Wraps

DID YOU KNOW?

CELIAC DISEASE IS NOW AT THE CENTER-STAGE OF THE SCIENTIFIC WORLD. THE PAST DECADE HAS BEEN VERY EXCITING AND PRODUCTIVE IN TERMS OF DIAGNOSTICS AND UNDERSTANDING THE BIOLOGY OF CELIAC DISEASE. WHILE GLUTEN-FREE DIET IS THE BEST MODE OF TREATMENT, MANY OTHER TARGETS FOR CONTROL OF THE IMMUNE-PATHOGENESIS OF CELIAC DISEASE ARE NOW ACTIVELY EXPLORED, SOME OF THEM HAVE REACHED EVEN PHASE 2 AND PHASE 3 CLINICAL TRIALS.

Quoted from:
17th International Celiac Disease Symposium in New Delhi, India

Best Gluten Free Vacation Destinations

10th Annual Gluten-Free Awards:

1st Place Winner: Walt Disney World

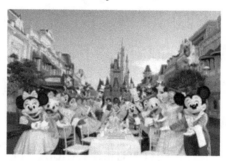

2nd Place Winner: Portland, OR

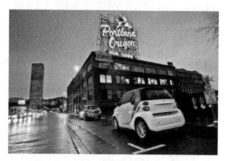

3rd Place Winner: Italy

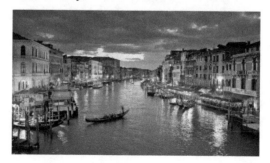

Other Great Vacation Locations:

New York City

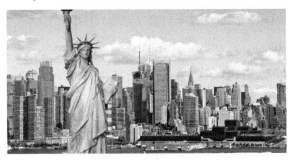

Royal Caribbean Cruises

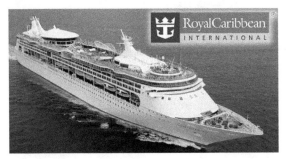

Disneyland, CA

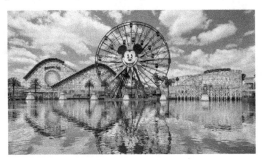

London, England

Grand Hyatt Kauai Resort & Spa

Disney Cruises

Sandals

Best Gluten Free Website

10th Annual Gluten-Free Awards:

1st Place Winner: gfJules.com

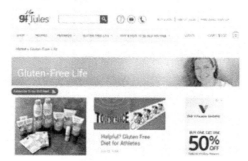

2nd Place Winner: Celiac.org

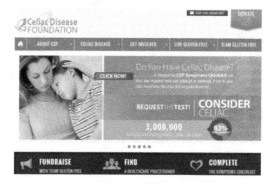

3rd Place Winner: What The Fork Food Blog

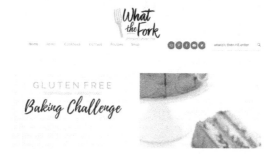

Other Great Gluten Free Websites:

Gluten Free Watch Dog

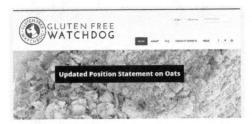

Celiac and the Beast

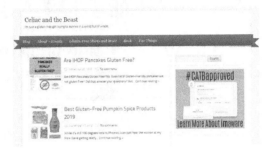

Gluten Free Follow Me.com

Gluten Dude

Gluten Free Travel Site

Cure Celiac Disease.org

Gluten Free Globetrotter

Gluten Free RN

Grain Changer

GlutenfreeGlobalicious

Jenna Drew.com

BuenQamino

Gluten-Free-Way.com

DID YOU KNOW?

AFTER BEING WELL RECOGNIZED IN EUROPE AND AMERICA, CELIAC DISEASE IS NOW GETTING RECOGNIZED IN ASIAN COUNTRIES. IT IS PREDICTED THAT THE NUMBER OF PATIENTS WITH CELIAC DISEASE IN ASIA MAY SURPASS THE NUMBERS PRESENT IN REST OF THE WORLD.

Quoted from:
17th International Celiac Disease Symposium in New Delhi, India

CELIAC SURVEY

We polled over 400 people with celiac disease
with the intent to make you feel not so alone.

Do you feel alone living the gluten free lifestyle?

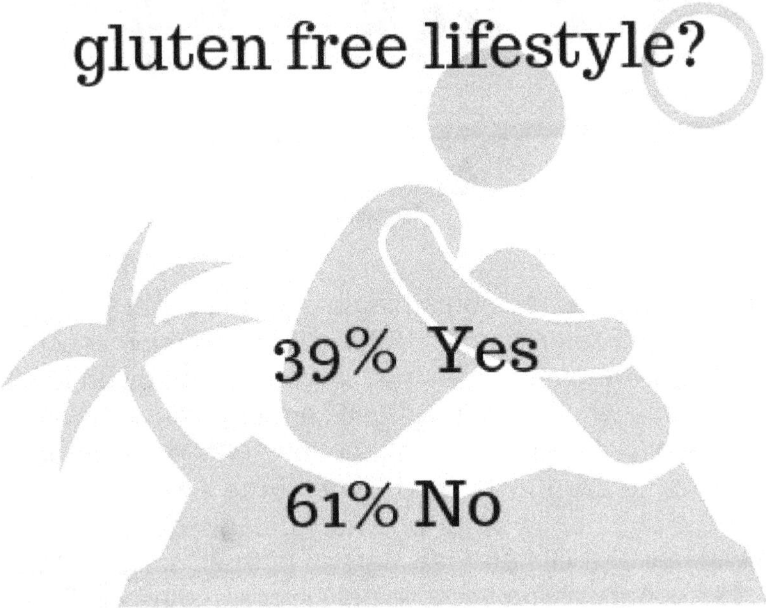

39% Yes

61% No

Presented by The 2020 Gluten Free Buyers Guide

YOU'RE NOT ALONE

Gluten Free Person of the Decade

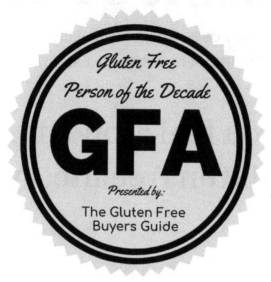

I always envisioned something big for our tenth year hosting the Gluten Free Awards.   After a brainstorming session with the team, we came up with a ten-year award given to somebody who has made significant contributions to the community, voted by the community.   We added a new category to the 10th Annual Gluten Free Awards ballot and had the community write who they thought deserved an award for The Gluten Free Person of the Decade.   With 3,937 people voting you can only imagine the long list of names that came up, however, one person stood out, gaining the largest number of votes.

I was excited to share the news with her but what do you say to somebody who won an award for a decade worth of work? I have known her for nine of these years and started to recall the great things she had accomplished and couldn't agree more with the voters.   I intend to share a summary of her decade's work but know it won't do it any justice.   She has truly moved the needle for those of us needing a gluten free diet to survive. I am honored to present "The Gluten Free Person of the Decade" to Jules Shepard.

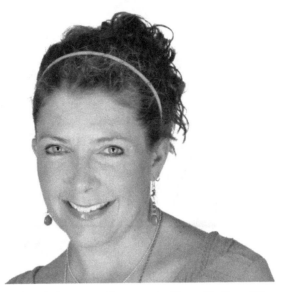

A former domestic violence attorney with a Celiac Disease diagnosis in 1999 Jules Shepard would not settle for substandard products. For two years she set out to perfect her own flour blend, a much-needed product for an avid baker. She didn't intend to create a business around this amazing product, but word quickly spread and has now sold over one million pounds of her fabulous flour. She first sold products under the name"Jules Gluten Free", but a business deal gone terribly bad forced her to start from scratch and sell exclusively as a new company, gfJules®.

gfJules® has now spread into multiple product lines and has received several Gluten Free Awards. Jules Shepard is not only an award-winning entrepreneur she is an advocate. To gain FDA attention during a gluten free labeling stall, she built a world record, 11-foot-tall, one-ton gluten free cake. News of the world record cake spread like whipped frosting across the nation and gained the FDAs' attention. Gluten free food labeling ultimately changed in 2014 and we have

Jules to thank for her ability to poke and prod the government to finally act.

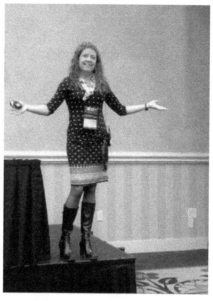

She acts as an expert witness for the gluten free community and ABC and Time Magazine uses her for article advice. She travels thousands of miles each year attending industry trade shows, hosting cooking classes and speaking.   She writes several magazine articles each year and maintains a very popular blog (gfjules.com/gluten-free-life/).   Jules is also an active mom, wife and caregiver.   She is a giving member of the gluten free community and is always thinking about "the other person".   In fact, when we discussed her award over the phone, she felt Dr. Alessio Fasano should have received it.

Jules, on behalf of the gluten free community, thank you for all that you do. We wouldn't be where we are today without you.

Gluten Free Product Registration

By submitting your products into The Gluten Free Awards (GFA), you are automatically entering products into the Annual Gluten Free Buyers Guide. There are only 10 slots available in each category and we limit brands to 3 submissions per category. If you are a marketer representing multiple brands, this typically will not apply. Slots can fill quickly so we recommend submitting your registration ASAP. The absolute deadline for registration is August 22nd however, we cannot guarantee you that the category is already full.

"How do I get into the Gluten Free Awards?"

How it works:

1. Fill out the registration form by adding the quantities and product names.

(A free half page ad is given for every 5 products or full-page ad for 10 products.)

2. If wanted, add additional ad space to registration.

3. Email the registration form to Jayme@GlutenFreeBuyersGuide.com

4. We will follow up with a confirmation and invoice.

If you have any questions call customer support at 828-455-9734

"Wait, I have tons of questions still"

Most common questions:

Q: I am having a hard time understanding how to submit or products.

A: Using this Registration Form will help. If lost, don't hesitate to call or email. 828-455-9734

Q: What are the image specs you need?

A: Our graphic team just needs images that are PDF, JPEG or PNG at 300 dpi or greater. The team will normally resize images based on the publishing media. Normally the product pictures and descriptions from your website will work just fine.

Full Page Ad Size 384 by 576 px

Half Page Ad Size 384 by 288 px

Q: Is there a word count for product descriptions?

A: No, we normally don't use product descriptions just product names and images.

Q: If we submit 10 products do we get 1 free full-page ad and 2 free half page ads?

A: Sorry, please choose one or the other. You can always purchase additional ad space.

Q: Can we run a full-page ad without entering the awards program?

A: Yes.

Q: Do we need to send you product samples?

A: No. The gluten-free community votes for your products.

Q: Will we be in the guide if we don't win an award?

A: Yes, all products submitted will be visible as nominees.

Q: Can we use the GFA Nominee and Winner Badge on our product packaging, website and other related media?

A: Yes, we highly recommend using the badges to differentiate your products from the rest. If you happen to need higher resolution images don't hesitate to ask. Read our media terms here.

Need to talk about your order or have questions? Give us a call.

828-455-9734

or email

Josh@GlutenFreeBuyersGuide.com

From our family to yours, have a happy and healthy gluten free lifestyle.

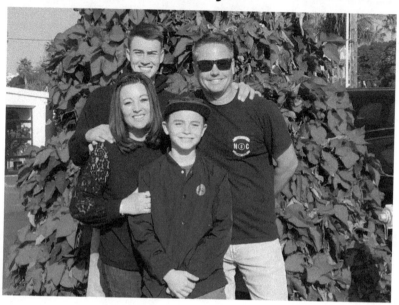

The Schieffer Family

Josh (Dad with Celiac) Chief Marketing Officer

Jayme (Mom) VP Operations

Blake (19)

Jacob (15 Celiac)

Keep up to date with us, the awards, and future buyer guides at GlutenFreeBuyersGuide.com